1979

Contents

Contents

Preface

Infanticide, for the purposes of the present volume, may be defined as the wilful destruction of an infant through exposure, starvation, strangulation, smothering, poisoning, or through the use of some lethal instrument or weapon. It is also useful to distinguish between malevolent and benevolent infanticide, where the latter is understood to be an act whose purpose is to benefit or help, or at least not to injure, the one who dies. This book, in the main, is devoted to the question of benevolent infanticide. Its primary purpose is to understand what conditions, if any, warrant allowing or inducing the death of a seriously defective infant. More generally, the debate is concerned with two questions: What are the limits of the value of life? And what moral, legal, or other kinds of protection should be provided for the most helpless and vulnerable of all human beings?

The book is divided into four parts. Part One is devoted to religio-ethical questions. Joseph Fletcher discusses the relationship of suicide, allocide (proxy suicide), euthanasia, and infanticide. He argues that abortion and infanticide can be justified when the consequence is that the good gained outweighs the evil—that neither abortion nor infanticide is as such immoral. Immanuel Jakobovits, on the other hand, maintains that all life has intrinsic, absolute, and infinite value; that a physically or mentally deficient human being has exactly the same value as any completely normal person; and that under no circumstances would Judaism countenance the killing of an infant already born. E.-H. W. Kluge briefly describes the nature of the right to life and personhood. He maintains that most infants are persons, and that unless their right to life is superseded by the rights of other persons, or their status as persons and particular situation combine to require euthanasia, to kill them is to commit murder. For Richard Brandt the fundamental question is neither that of personhood nor human rights. The fundamental question is whether rational or fully informed persons would, in view of the total consequences, support a moral code for a society in which they expected to live, with one, or another, provision on this matter. After discussing various problems including those of moral duty, consent, and quality of life, Brandt concludes that, since the lives of some defective newborns are destined to be bad on the whole, it would be a favor to them if their lives were terminated.

Part Two is concerned with anthropological, psychological, and medical issues. Laila Williamson compares different cultures in an attempt to determine the extent and nature of the various practices of infanticide. Her findings indicate that infanticide has been practiced on every continent and by people of every cultural complexity; that infanticide is seldom an expression of cruel or violent feelings; and that the reasons for infanticide have been overwhelmingly economic and demographic. By way of contrast, Brandt Steele's paper describes some of the main features of the psychology of infanticide related to maltreatment. Dr. Steele reminds us that the conservative estimate of two thousand deaths resulting from maltreatment each year in the United States is only a small fraction of the enormous amount of irreparable physical and emotional damage caused by prevalent patterns of violent, unloving care of small children.

Many thinkers distinguish between so-called active euthanasia (the situation in which the agent does something to end life "actively") and passive euthanasia (the situation where the physician or other agent "lets nature take its course"). More often than not, traditional or conservative writers maintain that only passive euthanasia is morally permissible. Others argue that the distinction is conceptually dubious or morally irrelevant. Peter Black's paper addresses itself to the latter problem. It asks and affirmatively answers the question whether a difference between killing and letting die can be morally supported.

Raymond Duff and Anthony Shaw are primarily concerned about

the problem of infant care and termination of life decision procedures in hospital nurseries. According to Duff, our attitudes and practices—regarding who shall live or die and how—must be revised if we truly care about people. "If caring is to be optimal," he concludes, "coercive living, like coercive dying, has no place among our choices." Anthony Shaw explores the question of who should die and who will decide. Not only does he describe the results and implications of a national survey of pediatricians and pediatric surgeons, but he is one of the first physicians to clearly recognize the importance of the concept of having a meaningful life.

Part Three deals with legal questions. The basic issue here is the premise that life, whatever its form, nature, or content, is necessary and always a good and that death, or any event that hastens death, is always and necessarily an evil and should be illegal. In essence, Glanville Williams and Arval Morris argue that laws prohibiting mercy infanticide are not necessary and often harmful, while Leonard Weber maintains that such laws are necessary if we are going to preserve our social health and welfare as a people. The general discussion is unusually rich and fruitful. Among other things, it illustrates that utilitarianism (or perhaps more accurately, consequentualism) does not necessarily commit one to any particular legal position.

Part Four raises some of the most formidable of ideological and philosophical questions. What is the preferable stance that ought to be taken towards suffering? Is it irrational to prefer blank annihilation to a life which is irrevocably meaningless or which, in balance, is on the side of torture? And under what conditions would a beneficent rational society allow its members to voluntarily leave off living? John Donnelly opens the discussion with a paper on the problem of suffering. He suggests that the term "suffering" be more carefully distinguished from the term "pain." That "suffering" is more properly applied to periods of intense pain or displeasure or mental anguish, and the consequent frustration of some basic (nontrivial) human needs and goals. Following Kierkegaard, he maintains that suffering often has great instrumental worth; that since suffering brings us closer to God, the meaning of life is contained in suffering; and that the true Christian, the true religious, will choose and relish suffering. In her paper "If There's Life, Make It Worth Living," Karen Metzler appears to maintain that, because we abhor suffering, ugliness, and imperfection, we have a tendency to kill or mistreat defective children. In the former case we deprive them of the right to taste and enjoy life; in the latter we deprive them of love, care, and concern: the very foundations of a quality life. Metzler urges us to change our attitude, to behave more lovingly, and thereby greatly enhance the quality of the lives of the handicapped. Joseph Margolis discusses a related issue. He begins his paper with an analysis of the questions, "when is life no longer worthwhile, no longer worth living?" and then sketches several arguments. Three of the most important conclusions seem to be (a) that there is no way of discovering by any familiar independent inquiry whether we are forbidden to end life or when it is correct to end life, apart from our own sensibilities and interests; (b) that judging that it is better to die rather than to live on does not entail that life is not worthwhile or no longer worth living or worthless; and (c) that the genus of such determinate forms of acting as suicide, murder, euthanasia, and the like must rest on moral criteria that cannot be reduced to or replaced by technical criteria of any sort. Stephen Nathanson is concerned with the relation of rationality and the value of life. He critically evaluates two major positions. According to Nathanson, the nihilistic perspective is inappropriate because it tends to overlook the difference between the question of what a purely rational being (in the sense of one possessing only cognitive powers) would necessarily choose and the question of what a rational being who possesses needs and various interests would necessarily choose. The Rawlsian analysis of value, on the other hand, has considerable merit. Nevertheless, Nathanson suggests that it cannot settle the controversy concerning the choice of death in situations where a person can make no choice for himself. The purpose of my own contribution is to determine whether or not it is morally permissible to end a human life if that life is meaningless; and, more generally, to determine how much voluntary death we want to allow—where, and when, and of what kind. The conclusions reached are that, given a theory of utilitarianism in which beneficence is the architectonic positive duty, there are circumstances involving altruism, imminent natural death, and meaningless existence in which we should allow people to die by their own hands or with the assistance of others; that death is not an injury for human beings when we allow their lives to end or put them to death even if they cannot—or have failed to—state their preferences if they are living a completely meaningless life and that state of affairs is irreparable and irreversible; and that death may be the best thing when life is too awful.

With the exception of Glanville Williams's paper, which is a revision of part of Chapter 1 of *The Sanctity of Life and the Criminal Law* (Knopf, 1957), all contributions appear here for the first time. An attempt has been made to represent contrasting points of view. However, since the majority of papers express the belief that some form of active voluntary death or benevolent infanticide may be permissible, there is no exact balance of pro and con positions. The volume is a prolegomena. Some papers were invited to draw attention to neglected issues, or to provide some desirable nonphilosophical perspective. But for various reasons—and much to my regret—many important problems have been omitted. There is a need for a better understanding of the history of infanticide, the psychology of the benevolent termination of life, the attitudinal requirements of parenthood, the extent to which a rational society must learn to accept suffering, how we ought to choose the ends of life, and why we can not morally require greater beneficence—to name some of the more salient problems. I claim for the included materials only that they serve to raise a good number of the great questions, not that they represent anything approaching an exhaustive survey of questions or of answers.

I am grateful to Sidney Hook for his good advice and almost infinite patience. One person, Barbara Bergstrom, not only read the entire draft and made many helpful suggestions, but also assisted in the proofreading, preparation of the final manuscript, and index.

In dedicating this book to my children I wish to indicate not only my deepest affection for them but also my appreciation for their zest, a vitality that has added significantly to my understanding of the great beauty and value of life.

M.K.

Fredonia, New York
July 1978

I.
RELIGIOETHICAL ISSUES

Joseph Fletcher

Infanticide and the Ethics of Loving Concern

The question whether infanticide is ever justifiable, and if so when, can be approached more appreciatively if we begin by locating infanticide on the total map of induced death, that is to say, of death humanly intended and contrived. Therefore, I shall first look at the moral variants in a spectrum of the different ways we might take to induce death, and then focus on infanticide in particular.

In what follows we will be looking primarily at dying when it is chosen or elected in the sick room, which might be called medical euthanasia; I will prescind from such practices as vendetta, military life taking, capital punishment, mortal risk-benefit choices, and other ways of assuming control over life and death—other kinds of human decisions not to leave death to "natural" causes. *The Oxford English Dictionary* defines euthanasia (literally "good death" or what medieval philosophers called *bene mori*) this way: "In recent use: the action of inducing a gentle and easy death." Several variables arise between medical and non-medical situations, even though the constants are equally important. In our present society, however, the problem is more commonly posed in the context of medical care and treatment.

The moral problems of suicide and allocide are, of course, not new. Nevertheless, they are taking a new shape recently because of advances in medical capabilities, especially in resuscitation and life-support technologies. Once upon a time the typical problem in serious life-threatening illnesses was to find a way to prolong life, but often now the problem is how long and how much to do so, particularly when we find we are prolonging dying rather than living, "saving" biological life at the expense of human life.

LOCATING INFANTICIDE

My premise will be that induced death, as such, may not be condemned categorically, and that truly rational ethical issues only arise when responsible moral agents set about determining answers to operational questions—who, why, what, when, and how. It is unreasonable ethically to say that all acts of euthanasia are wrong, just as it would be to say that none are.

Another premise is that what is good and right for a person when he does it for himself, e.g., suicide, is just as good and right, and for the same reasons, when it is done for him by proxy (i.e., allocide). Thus the English law which decriminalizes self-administered euthanasia but continues to outlaw it when it is carried out by others, such as physicians, nurses, paramedics, or a member of the family, at the subject's request or with his agreement, is logically untenable.

The most significant ethical discrimination we make when we evaluate intended and induced dying ("elective death") is between voluntary and involuntary cases. This would, at least, be true for those with whom freedom of choice is a highly important element of personal integrity—a first-order value. The "right-to-die" is therefore taken ordinarily to mean one's right to choose one's own death, rather than any right (at least ordinarily) to choose death for somebody else.

Voluntary dying is chosen consciously by the subject, whether in the event or prior to it. An example would be fulfilling the wishes of patients that treatment be stopped when to do anything more would be fatuous. Their wishes might be expressed either at that time or recorded earlier in a living will. Involuntary dying would be exemplified by an accident victim's death on the operating table, or when a comatose patient's treatment is stopped because to continue would be pointless and cruel—the decision being made without the patient's consent and without any knowledge of his preference, past or present. The difference hangs on the factor of consent.

Euthanasia, however, poses not one but four critical distinctions. Its form may vary not only as to (1) consent (voluntary or involuntary); but also as to (2) whether the method used to end the patient's life is by a positive act or by omitting life-preserving treatment (direct or indirect); (3) whether the agent of the action is the subject himself or somebody else (active or passive); and (4) whether the patient's condition is terminal or nonterminal—i.e., whether or not death has been determined to be imminent.

Direct euthanasia is death induced by doing something that entails the patient's death as an immediate consequence. Instances would be the patient taking a highly toxic drug such as potassium cyanide, or the physician's administering it, or somebody removing an endotracheal tube from a patient with pulmonary arrest. Euthanasia is indirect when something is done that foreseeably results in death as a "subsequence" but not the direct consequence. Such would be a patient's refusal to eat, or if he (or another) disconnected intravenous inserts for hyperalimentation (i.e., starving the patient to death). This direct-indirect distinction has to do, in short, with whether the relation between cause and effect is immediate or not, i.e., whether the foreseeable result of the action follows at once from the act or only after a series of effects set in train by the primary action.

A pathetic case illustrating the direct-indirect phase of infanticide occurred some years ago at the Johns Hopkins Hospital in Baltimore; it has had a wide follow-up discussion, based on a film about it circulated for teaching purposes. A newborn had all the stigmata of Down's syndrome and the parents therefore refused consent to the corrective surgery needed to remove a duodenal atresia and thus open up the infant's food tract and save it from death.

The physicians in charge believed that direct euthanasia is wrong but that doing it indirectly, though undesirable, was morally tolerable. Hoping that it would die of dehydration and starvation in three or four days, they wheeled it off into a corner where it lay dying for fifteen days, not three or four. Some form of direct termination would have been far more merciful as far as the infant, nurses, parents, and some of the physicians were concerned. In that case indirect was morally worse than direct—if, as I and most of us would contend, the good and the right are determined by human wellbeing. Indirect euthanasia did no good at all in that case, but lots of evil.

The third distinction, between active and passive, has to do with whether an act of euthanasia is done by the patient or by somebody else. It is active when the subject (patient) does it, for example, by taking an overdose of a barbiturate or opiate. It is passive when another person does it for the subject, whether directly (e.g., closing down a patient's lungs with a specific for pulmonary paralysis) or indirectly (e.g., removing the support provided by a respirator). We have already suggested that there is no ethical difference between active and passive ways of inducing death. The only difference is in the agent, which makes it suicide or allocide, but this is instrumental, not intentional. Either way the patient's death is the end being sought, whether the patient or some other person brings it about. If the patient's release from an irreversibly painful and hopeless existence is contrived for him instead of by him, no onus lies on the agent unless it lies on the patient too.

By the same reasoning, direct and indirect euthanasia are morally alike, on a par. As I have put it elsewhere, "It is morally evasive and disingenuous to suppose that we can condemn or disapprove positive acts of care and compassion but in spite of that approve negative strategies to achieve exactly the same purpose."[1] Kant was on sound ground to insist that if we will the end, we will the means. Purposive acts of commission are morally no different from acts of omission that have the same goal. A decision not to open an imperforate anus in a trisomy-18 newborn is "mercy killing" as surely as if they used a poison pellet. Not eating is suicide as surely as jumping off the Eiffel Tower; it just takes longer.

Our fourth and last distinction is between terminal and nonterminal cases. A patient is terminal if he is going to die of his present condition no matter what treatment is given; an example would be the man with amyotrophic lateral sclerosis in Dr. I. S. Cooper's novel, *It's Hard to Leave When the Music's Playing.*[2] A nonterminal case would be one in which death would not be expected from any present pathology; e.g., a person who hangs himself because his life, as such, does not seem worth living.

In short, euthanasia has significantly different forms. It may be voluntary or involuntary, direct or indirect, active or passive, a response to terminal illness or to some other condition. A number of combinations and permutations of these variances is to be met with every day in the realities of dying, as human beings strive to control dying for human or humane reasons. Some of these differences, however, are without much, if any, ethical weight.

INFANTICIDE

Infanticide is the induced death (euthanasia) of infants. Because of their various deficits, when death comes to infants it is necessarily involuntary. Whether it comes naturally or by human design it happens without the subject's knowledge or consent. Knowledge and consent are impossible—as impossible for neonates as for fetuses when abortion is considered. It is reasonable, indeed, to describe infanticide as postnatal abortion, which is what it obviously was in the South Pacific when Robert Louis Stevenson visited the atolls and found that the Polynesians practiced infanticide with newborns showing disabling birth diseases and defects. (Theirs was a situation of radically scarce resources, both economic and medical, and Stevenson's initial revulsion was set aside after a period of observation.)

Furthermore, infanticide is passive. An infant cannot put an end to its own life. This makes it allocide, not suicide. Its variables are only (1) with respect to the euthanasiast's choice of direct or indirect means; and (2) whether it is done within the context of terminal illness or some other adverse state.

Some writers have argued that a fetus is a person as truly as an infant is, and that therefore both abortion and infanticide are unjust killing (murder). This argument has as its premise the rule that persons (human beings) ought never to elect or be elected to die by human initiatives. This universal negative or prohibition implies that death must always be imposed nonhumanly by God or nature or some other cosmic arbiter. It is a position with which we are familiar in classical Catholic moral theology and Protestant ethics (although not all theologians defend it), and in "pro-life" propaganda. Paul Ramsey has defended this view.[3] I have contended for the opposite position, i.e., that both abortion and infanticide can be justified if and when the good to be gained outweighs the evil—that neither abortion nor infanticide is as such immoral.[4] John Fletcher has tried to establish a middle position, arguing for the liceity of abortion but against infanticide.[5] He gives three reasons why infants are different from fetuses and should be differently treated: (1) a neonate has a separate existence, (2) tends to arouse parental feelings of attachment, and (3) is treatable. (Each of these things, however, is true of fetuses too.)

Another ground for opposing infanticide has been chosen by E-H.

W. Kluge.[6] His major premise is his belief or metaphysical assertion that an infant is a person, which he defines as any individual with not only an actual but a *potential* capacity for human self-awareness. His contention is that persons *qua* persons have a right to live—and that ethically this right may not be abridged. Because in his opinion a "structural potential" exists in fetuses (he fails to discriminate those cases in which the potential is not present), he assigns personal status to both fetuses and infants. He concludes: "Therefore infanticide is—to say the least—morally reprehensible. In fact, it is murder." (This appears to be an instance of the fallacy of the potential, i.e., arguing by prolepsis that the potential is the actual. Henry David Aiken calls this fallacy in this context "fetishism."[7])

Here we come to the crucial issue. Do persons, however defined, have an absolute or unqualified right to live? The courts have never found one, nor has jurisprudence. So-called human rights, as a term much employed in political rhetoric, are certain moral claims (e.g., to privacy, to property, liberty, and the like) that are ordinarily or commonly conceded. Street talk about "rights" ("I have a right to" such things as relief checks, free parking, health care, education, old age benefits, or whatever) means nothing more than an expression of belief, well or ill founded, that people *ought* to have certain things. However, all these claims are only relatively valid, whether they are or are not constitutionally formulated. At best they are only "prima facie." They are relative and not absolute for the sufficient reason that they can and often do cut across each other. Ethical problems are, when thoroughly examined, problems of relative choice among competing values or "goods," and to posit values at all entails priorities for making risk-benefit and gain-loss judgments. Hence the relativity of rights.

Kluge's real sting is in his tail. Not until the very last sentence of his discussion of infanticide does he come out of the closet and declare openly, "And if it is argued that this [condemnation of infanticide] depends on the further assumption that there are absolute values, I must unabashedly admit that this is something I hold to be the case."[8]

This means, if it means anything, that the life of persons, which he believes infants and fetuses to be, has an absolute value that cannot be relatively weighed by any moral scales to other competing values and dysvalues. It means that life, as such, is sacrosanct and taboo, no matter how much suffering and tragedy and deprivation might be the price.[9] Given this as his "bottom line," he (Kluge) could not cope with the decision making for an infant with 94.5 percent full-thickness, 92 percent to-tal-body burns and irreversible lung damage from smoke inhalation. Or, again, how could he make a judgment ethically about an infant with spina bifida cystica, plus a meningomyelocele and meningeal infection already widespread? Or about an infant born with retinoblastoma after slipping through the antenatal screen, when postoperative diagnosis shows that the surgical removal of its eyes has not stopped the spread of cancer?

If the life of these infants, such as it is, is sacrosanct as far as human initiatives are concerned, they would have to suffer—according to the taboo ethic—until they died "naturally" or until "God called them" out of life. If life is absolutely good, unconditionally good, we cannot talk about quality of life, since in common use the phrase requires us to be open to judging the quality of life itself, as well as making quality judgments on things within the ambiance of life. As the Jesuit theologian, R. A. McCormick, once put it, ethical reasoning collapses when anybody says, "There is no such thing as a life not worth living."[10]

The rejoinder to Kluge and others like him is that they have misplaced the debate. Careful and candid analysis will show that deciding whether and when an infant is a person is not the determinative question.[11] The right one is, "Can a person's life ever be ended ethically?" (Kluge compromises his taboo by allowing one exception—killing in self-defense.) It all turns on the issue of whether the value of a human life is absolute or relative.[12] It is this "metaethical" question which lies at the heart of the disagreement about infanticide. We could accept Kluge's thesis that fetuses are persons and still justify abortion and infanticide in some cases, because, in a given case, to prolong life would be to engender more evil than good. This tragic situation occurs frequently in perinatal medicine, even though its frequency is not great statistically. It is Kluge's second premise (that we may not take a person's life) that is rejectable, whether or not we accept his first premise (that fetuses and infants are persons.)[13]

Pediatricians or others who would sometimes justify letting a newborn die, or even helping a newborn die, would do so on value grounds. Life itself would be only one value among values, even though a high-order one, and therefore some infants' lives (like some lives in any other age group) might properly be sacrificed on the principle of proportionate good. No undeclared premises are hiding behind the discussion in this essay. It is based on ethical relativism—i.e., situational or contextual relativism, not cultural relativism. This is my mode of approach to the ethics of induced death in general and infanticide in particular.

To contend that there are cases in which it is good, and therefore right, to induce the end of a person's life obviously assigns the first-order value to human wellbeing, either by maximizing happiness or minimizing suffering; it assigns value to human life rather than to merely being alive. On this view it is better to be dead than to suffer too much or to endure too many deficits of human function. In this mode of ethical reasoning the criterion of obligation is caring or kindness or loving concern—various terms have been used to denote it.[14] Its basic value stance is that we ought to do whatever promotes wellbeing and reduces suffering, and therefore, if ending a life is judged to do so, so be it.

William Frankena has classified my ethics as "modified act agapism," which simply means that loving concern for human beings comes first, before rules of conduct.[15] As Frankena shows, it is a form of utilitarianism and consequentialist ethical decision making. The only "rule" it follows consistently is to do whatever offers the most human benefit, and on this basis we would sometimes save lives, sometimes end them (directly or indirectly, actively or passively).

In another place citing various philosophical discussions, Frankena rashly and arbitrarily says that Henry Sidgwick, William Temple, and I all assume that belief in the "sanctity of life" means holding life to be absolute and inviolable, but, in fact, all three of us accept the distinction Frankena draws between *absolute* respect for life (not, however, sanctifying it) and "*qualified* respect for human life"—which last Frankena and the rest of us endorse, all alike.[16]

Loving concern ("agape") is a standard of good and evil that could be validated in either a theistic or a humanistic belief system. A theist might, of course, believe that God forbids infanticide by a rule, perhaps along with other things such as adultery or baking bread on Sundays. On the other hand, he might believe that the divine will or command is only that we do the most loving thing possible in a given situation, leaving it to the moral agent to decide what that is. Likewise, a humanist might decide that ending infants' lives is in general inhumane and therefore ought never to be done (as with some rule utilitarians),[17] or he might hold instead that we should seek to optimize human wellbeing in every case, thus allowing for infanticide sometimes (as in act utilitarianism).

If one's standard of the good is human wellbeing, and one's duty or obligation is to seek to increase it wherever possible, with a consequent willingness to save lives sometimes and end them sometimes, then it will follow that infanticide is acceptable (sometimes). If one's standard is a divine will or other cosmic authority (e.g., Natural Law), one could still accept infanticide, depending on whether the divine will is believed to be expressed in universal and absolute rules (such as we can find in revealed codes), or in a general command to be loving (beneficent, kind, humane, et cetera) with flexibility as to the variables in particular cases.

In fact, the differences between religious ethics and ethical autonomy do not determine the issue of the ethics of infanticide. The only real issue is whether concern for persons in hopeless misery ranks higher or lower than taboo.

Notes

1. Joseph Fletcher, "Ethics and Euthanasia," *American Journal of Nursing*, 73 (April 1973): 670-675.
2. I. S. Cooper, *It's Hard to Leave When the Music's Playing* (New York: W. W. Norton & Co., 1977).
3. Paul Ramsey, "Abortion," *The Thomist* 37 (1973): 174-226.
4. Ramsey, "Abortion," pp. 174-226.
5. John Fletcher, "Abortion, Euthanasia, and Care of Defective Newborns," *The New England Journal of Medicine* 292 (January 9, 1975): 75-78.
6. Eike-Henner W. Kluge, *The Practice of Death* (New Haven, Conn.: Yale University Press, 1975), pp. 207-209.
7. Henry David Aiken, "Life and the Right to Life," in *Ethical Issues in Human Genetics*, ed. Bruce Hilton et al. (New York: Plenum Press, 1973), p. 182.
8. Later on Kluge says that although there are absolute rules, nobody has yet identified them, and this he promises to do some day. Kluge, *Practice of Death*, pp. 242-244.
9. As Barbara Kellum and others have shown, even in the religious era of medieval England, infanticide, like abortion, was regarded as only a venial sin, not mortal. Thomas of Cobham's penitential said that if an infant was disposed of by its mother's own hand, it was a venial sin on a par with overlaying, and a refusal to nurse an infant was also. For a summary account, see Cyril Means, "The Phoenix of Abortional Freedom," 17 *New York Law Forum* 335 (1971).
10. R. A. McCormick, "To Save or Let Die: the Dilemma of Modern Medicine," *Journal of the American Medical Association* 229 (July 8, 1974): 172-176.
11. Michael Tooley also focusses on the problem of *when* a neonate acquires "a serious right to life," which he concludes is decisive for both fetuses and infants. But the right question is something else, i.e., Is this right absolute, no matter how the right itself is established? See Tooley's "Abortion and Infanticide," *Philosophy and Public Affairs* 2 (1972): 37-65.
12. Aiken, "Life and the Right to Life," shows why the right to life is "not only conditional but contingent."
13. He cannot justify an absolute taboo on humane or humanistic grounds. It must presumably be supported by a cosmic authority, God or Mother Nature, established by revelation or metaphysics, but whatever it is, he keeps it secret and undeclared.
14. Bentham and Mill called it utility. Marvin Kohl calls it "reasonable kindness" in his *The Morality of Killing* (New York: Humanities Press, and London: Peter Owen, 1974). In my own language it is called loving concern (Joseph Fletcher, *Situation Ethics* [Philadelphia: Westminster Press, 1966]).

15. See William Frankena, *Ethics*, 2nd ed. (Englewood Cliffs, N.J.: Prentice-Hall, 1973), pp. 36, 55-57.

16. William Frankena, "The Ethics of Respect for Life," *Respect for Life in Medicine, Philosophy and Law*, ed. O. Temkin, W. K. Frankena, and S. H. Kadish (Baltimore: Johns Hopkins University Press, 1976), pp. 32-33.

17. Rule utilitarianism could theoretically set up an opposite norm or rule, that it is right to practice infanticide in certain kinds or classes of situations.

Immanuel Jakobovits

Jewish Views on Infanticide

The word "infanticide" as "the crime of murdering an infant after its birth, perpetrated by or with the consent of its parents, especially the mother" entered English usage in 1789.[1] But in English law it did not feature as a specific offense, distinct from ordinary murder or manslaughter, until it became a modern felony by statute in 1922 (modified in 1938). This holds a woman guilty of infanticide if she kills her child while it is under the age of twelve months, and while the balance of her mind is disturbed from the effects of giving birth. Neither the father nor any other person can be charged with this offense.[2] Of course, we are here concerned with the wider and more popular meaning of the term as the killing of an infant, especially in cases of grave congenital abnormalities, whoever commits the act.

In Hebrew there is no equivalent for infanticide. Such an act, as we understand it and as widely practiced in pagan society, is simply unknown both as a phenomenon in Jewish history and as a distinct rubric in Jewish law. Significantly, it is only under the heading of *"Kiddush HaShem"* ("Sanctification of the Divine name," i.e., martyrdom) that any reference to the deliberate killing of children by Jews can be found in works covering the entire gamut of Jewish life and thought, like the *Encyclopedia Judaica*[3] and S. W. Baron's massive *A Social and Religious History of the Jews.*[4]

Jewish law makes no distinction whatever between infants and adults in their claim to life. It expressly construes the verse "And he that smites any human life [mortally] shall surely be put to death" (Lev. 24:17) to include the murder of minors.[5] As codified by Maimonides,[6] murder is culpable as a capital offense "whether one kills an adult or a one-day-old child." The title to life is absolute, and equal to that of any other person, from the moment of birth, that is, the emergence of the head (or the greater part of the body) from the birth-canal. Prior to that moment, in the event of a mortal conflict between mother and child, and in the absence of any means to save the mother except by destroying her unborn child, one may (indeed, one must) do so, "since her life takes precedence over its life"; but if a possibly fatal complication sets in from that moment, "one must not touch it, since one does not set aside one human life for the sake of another."[7]

The only exception to this rule is of little, if any, relevance to our subject. The killing of a one-day-old child is punishable as murder only if it was carried to term and delivered after a full nine-months' pregnancy; otherwise it is not considered as definitely viable until it has passed the first thirty days of life. Accordingly, unless a full-term pregnancy can be proven beyond doubt (e.g., by the parents' separation for nine complete months), a child dying within thirty days, whether by violence or from natural causes, is presumed to have been a "miscarriage" (i.e., a non-viable birth). The killer of such a child is not liable to capital punishment,[8] nor are the normal mourning regulations to be observed upon its death.[9] This exemption also extends to death ensuing *after* the first thirty days, if the child was definitely born in the eighth month of pregnancy (which was considered to render it incapable of long-term survival) or if it was delivered in a maimed state.[10]

This reservation does not, however, imply that it is permitted to kill infants in these categories. Such an act is merely reduced from murder to noncapital homicide, as are certain other forms of causing death, such as by starvation or suicide,[11] or the killing of a fatally injured person.[12] These cases, though they cannot be tried before a human court, still constitute bloodshed for which the offender is accountable before the heavenly tribunal.

In practice, the presumption of nonviability, as defined above, affects the attitude to abortion rather than to infanticide. For instance, as we have seen, whilst an abortion is indicated by any hazard to the mother's life, a child must not be sacrificed for the sake of the mother *during* parturition once its head, or the greater part of its body, has been delivered. But what would be the verdict in such a situation—say, a breech birth endangering the mother because the child's head cannot be safely extracted—when the alternative to saving the mother at the expense of the child would be the death of both? In that event, it has been argued, the value of the child's life, though in principle equal to that of the mother or any other person, is still compromised by the doubt about its viability until it has lived for at least thirty days, to the extent that its inviolability does not outweigh the loss of both lives.[13] Similarly, this consideration may also apply to the abortion of fetuses shown to be afflicted with Tay-Sachs disease by an amniotic fluid test (amniocentesis) early in pregnancy. Rabbinic opinions are still divided on the right to resort to abortion in order to prevent the birth of children likely to be born with grave congenital defects.[14] But at least one permissive view is inclined to sanction the operation upon a positive diagnosis of Tay-Sachs, since the disease invariably proves fatal within the first three or four years of life and the child, were it to be born, would therefore not be viable.[15]

But these modifications—limited, as they are, to interventions before or possibly during birth—clearly have no bearing on infanticide. Indeed, there is no source or authority in Jewish law to support any suggestion that some line can be drawn between infants and other persons in this respect. On the contrary, in dealing with the supreme sanctity of life and its inviolability, reference is always made to a one-day-old infant as the commencing age in the full title to life. This applies to the legal definition of murder, as we have seen, just as it features in the dictum of the Talmud on the preservation of human life taking precedence even over acts of reverence for the dead: "For a one-day-old child [that is dangerously ill] the Sabbath may be profaned. . . ; for David, King of Israel, once he is dead, the Sabbath must not be violated."[16] Echoing the same spirit at about the turn of the twelfth century, over a thousand years later, a famous Jewish moralist work asserted that one must rescue from the flames any living infant rather than the dead body of one's own father.[17]

Accordingly, although questions on infanticide submitted to rabbinic judgment or discussed in rabbinic writings are very scarce, the answer is invariably a categorical no, however serious the defects in the child concerned. Thus, the moralist work just mentioned refers to a ruling against terminating the life of an infant born with teeth and tail like an animal, counseling instead the removal of these features.[18] Early in the nineteenth century, a leading rabbi advised a questioner that it was forbidden to destroy a grotesquely misshapen child; to kill any being born of a human mother, even by starvation, constituted unlawful homicide.[19]

The issue was catapulted into world-wide prominence—and controversy—by the celebrated trial in November 1962 at Liège (Belgium) that acquitted a mother and other accomplices of guilt for the confessed killing of a thalidomide baby. The shock-waves of this *cause célèbre* spilt over into the rabbinic world as well. The verdict was denounced in an extensive study by a widely recognized scholar who argued: "The sole legitimate grounds for killing a fetus are the urgent needs of the mother and her healing, whereas in these circumstances the mother's [action is motivated by] self-love . . . , wrapped in a cloak of compassion for this unfortunate creature, and this cannot be called a necessity for the mother at all."[20] Under no circumstances, then, would Judaism countenance the killing of an infant already born, on these or any other grounds.

Jewish law, then, would treat infanticide at best like any other form of euthanasia. The act is not rendered more objectionable by the fact that the patient, being a newborn infant, cannot give his consent; for consent is quite immaterial to the condemnation of euthanasia. But neither is the offense mitigated by the tender age of the victim. All the considerations militating against any sanction of euthanasia apply equally to infanticide.

The Jewish objection to direct euthanasia is uncompromising. To quote again from the passage in the Code of Maimonides already referred to, "whether one kills a healthy person or a patient who approaches death, or even a dying person, one is liable to capital punishment."[21] True, the killer is exempt from this penalty if the victim was close to death through injuries inflicted by the hand of man (i.e., not for natural causes)[22] or definitely suffered from some inevitably fatal affliction.[23] But these again are technical reservations that affect the mode of punishment, or the offender's indictability, rather than the nature of the crime as an inexcusable act of bloodshed. And even this qualification, inconsequential as it is in our context, has no bearing on infanticide in cases where the infant's defect is not liable to prove fatal.

But this rigid attitude relates only to active euthanasia. However, there has lately been some debate in rabbinic writings on passive euthanasia, i.e., the withdrawal of treatment by artificial means or "heroic methods" in hopeless cases at the terminal stage, especially when accompanied by intense pain. While some authorities would not sanction the suspension of efforts to preserve life by all available means even under such conditions, others do not require the physician to prolong the agony in these cases by recourse to other than natural means.[24] Under carefully defined conditions and safeguards, these latter authorities, though not permitting the withholding of food (being a natural means to sustain life), would not deem it mandatory to administer antibiotics or to apply artificial respirators, for example, in the event of complications combining with a cancer condition in the final phase.

In similar circumstances, this severely limited sanction would obviously apply to infants, too. But physical or mental abnormalities as such, however extreme, would not qualify for inclusion in this concession, unless they definitely restricted the expectancy of life to a short while. Even then, it must be reiterated with every emphasis, any sanction would not extend to the withholding of normal care and feeding, let alone to any deliberate killing. It would only justify the suspension of artificial means to combat the mortal effects of complications, such as infections or critical injuries. Such nonintervention in the course of nature, however, could hardly be classified as infanticide.

From these purely legal affirmations proscribing infanticide in rather absolute terms, we may now enucleate the moral reasoning underlying them, including some reflections on the Jewish attitude to suffering in general.

Basic to the attitude of Judaism is, above all, the Jewish concept of, and commitment to, the sanctity of human life. As nature abhors a vacuum, so does Jewish law eschew vague generalities for the definition of moral and ethical norms, preferring precise, practical definitions instead. It therefore spells out the sanctity of life in very specific terms, attributing *infinite value* to every innocent life.

Infinity is indivisible. Any fraction of infinity remains *equally* infinite. Hence, if seventy years of life are of infinite worth, so is one year, one week, one day, or one hour of life. All are equally valuable and inviolable. And just as the time factor is irrelevant to the worth of life, being infinite, so is the health of a person. Once the principle of infinity is established, it follows that a physically or mentally deficient human being has exactly the same value as any completely normal person. "Half a human being" is no more reduced in value by reason of his incapacity than half of infinity is less than infinity. A human "vegetable" is unknown in the moral or legal vocabulary of Judaism. Where there is life, there may not always be hope; but there is always the spark of a uniquely precious soul.

The reason for insisting on this principle of infinity is as logically simple as it is morally compelling. The moment it is conceded that a lingering patient with, say, another hour to live can be dispatched because his life is practically worthless, it follows that another liable to die in two hours would have twice this still infinitesimal value, and this value would appreciate as the expectancy of life increases. Thus, a person who is likely to live for only another week would be worth less than one whose prognosis gives him another year.

This means that *all* human beings would no longer have an absolute, but merely a relative, value—relative to their expectancy of life, state of health, usefulness to society, or any other arbitrary criterion. Consequently, no two persons would be equal in value, and people would be graded into those of superior and inferior worth, leading directly and inescapably to the Nazi doctrine whereby millions of "inferior" beings were shoved into the gas chambers and ovens. Once a single brick is removed from the dam protecting the sanctity of all life, the entire dam is liable to collapse and every life is at risk.

Of course, since in the Jewish view, all life thus has an intrinsic, absolute, and infinite value, this is not merely a "thin-end-of-the-wedge" argument. The thin end itself is fatal, even without being followed by the full width of the wedge. Infanticide, even if practiced on a hopelessly deformed baby, becomes a crime identical to the killing of a healthy child or adult, because both acts involve the destruction of something equally and infinitely precious. But additonally, the fear lest the slightest modification of the homicide laws lead to graver excesses is real enough. From the killing of a malformed infant it is only one slippery step to the elimination of cripples or senile people in advanced stages of degeneration. From there, it is only one further step to the destruction of other "undesirables" burdening society.

Moreover, where is a morally defensible line to be drawn between legitimate and illegitimate infanticide? At birth, or within an hour, a day, a week, a month, or a year thereafter? And how serious must the disability be—at what minimum point is the child's anticipated I.Q. to be set, or the extent of a physical abnormality to be fixed, to warrant the forfeiture of its claim to life and some (or any) human value?

The whole notion of assessing human life by some arbitrary differential—instead of deeming its worth as beyond measure, unique, and transcending any utilitarian quantification or qualification—is utterly repugnant to Judaism. It is an affront to the cardinal teaching that every human being is created "in the Divine image."[25]

Judaism is certainly as remote from indifference to suffering as it is from unconcern with compassion. Despairing cries like Rachel's "Give me children, or else I die"[26] and Job's fierce challenges to God's justice in the face of affliction have rung down the centuries loud and long enough to belie the claim that suffering must be accepted with stoic resignation, let alone that it should be sought as an ideal, either for self-purification or for spiritual merits in the hereafter. All this mortifying asceticism is quite alien to the Jewish tradition.

To be sure, the agonies of life, when they have to be endured, can and do have ennobling effects, and the Talmud ascribes atoning powers to them.[27] That the tragedy of a defective child may open up otherwise inaccessible resources of selfless love and other spiritual virtues is not in question. Heart-warming cases of superb dedication, matchless affection, and sometimes even sublime happiness being generated out of the ordeal of caring for an incapacitated child hardly require documentation. Quite apart from the intrinsic worth of life, a supreme objective value of a cruelly afflicted being may well lie in the refining influence such a life exercises on those charged tenderly to protect it.

But the recognition of this incidental benefit, no doubt real enough in some instances, is still a far cry from the affirmation of suffering as an essential or desirable means to human perfection. On the contrary, Judaism always regarded suffering as a curse to be mitigated or avoided. Jewish theologians were never troubled by the use of chloroform at childbirth or of other analgesics at the approach of death as "flying in the face of Providence." Even martyrdom was sanctioned only for "the sanctification of the Divine Name," not for the purification of the soul or other human ends.[28]

It is the law, rather than the pain inflicted by nature, that must be accepted with resignation. And it is life, any human life, not happiness or the contribution to society, that outweighs all other values. Jewish law, deeply concerned to relieve pain and misery, readily modified some of its most sacred precepts, such as various Sabbath laws, when they conflict with this concern.[28] The religious duty to protect sentient beings from avoidable pain extends even to animals,[29] as indeed also to capital criminals; the anxiety for their freedom from suffering introduces the entire concept of "securing an easy death" into Talmudic legislation.[30]

But the one concession Jewish law cannot make is to purchase the relief of suffering at the cost of life itself. What it can and does do, however, when suffering and hardship exceed the bounds of tolerance, is to charge society with the responsibilities individuals can no longer bear on their own, by providing economic and institutional aid to reduce the burden of stricken families. The solution to the tragic problem of grossly handicapped children lies not in killing them, but in intensifying the social conscience and services of the community whose children they are.

Notes

1. *The Shorter Oxford English Dictionary* 3rd. ed., 2 vol. (New York: Oxford University Press, 1973), 1:998.
2. See Norman St. John-Stevas, *The Right to Life* (New York: Holt, Rinehart & Winston, 1963), p. 18.
3. See *Encyclopedia Judaica*, Index volume, s. v. "Infanticide" (1:525), referring to suicides of whole families and slaughter of children by parents to escape forced conversion, especially during the Crusades, in article on *"Kiddush Ha-shem"* (10:983).
4. Salo W. Baron, *A Social and Religious History of the Jews*, 2nd rev. and enl. ed. (New York: Columbia University Press, 1957), 4:144, in a similar reference to the Crusades. Baron also records "the undertone of legitimate envy in Tacitus' remark that the Jews 'take thought to increase their numbers; for they regard it as a crime to kill any lateborn [*agnatis*, not desired] child' " (2:219).
5. *Sanhedrin* 84b; see Rashi on Ex. 21:12; and Lev. 24:17.
6. *Hil. Rotze'ach*, 2:6.
7. *Oholot*, 7:6; Maim., *Hil. Rotze'ach*, 1:9; and *Shulchan Aruch, Choshen Mishpat*, 425:2. See more fully "Jewish Views on Abortion," in Jakobovits, *The Timely and the Timeless*, London, 1977, pp. 349ff.
8. *Hil. Rotze'ach*, 2:6.
9. *Hil. Evel*, 1:6-7.
10. Ibid., 1:8.
11. *Hil. Rotze'ach*, 2:2-3.
12. Ibid., 7-8.
13. Israel Lipschuetz, *Tif'eret Yisrael*, on *Oholot*, 7:6, *Boaz*, no. 10. For this and other sources, see Immanuel Jakobovits, *Jewish Medical Ethics*, rev. ed. (New York: Bloch, 1975) pp. 187ff.
14. Jakobovits, *Jewish Medical Ethics*, pp. 273ff.
15. L. Grossnass, responsa *Lev Aryeh*, 2:49. See Jakobovits, *Jewish Medical Ethics*, pp. 262ff; and Jakobovits, *The Timely and the Timeless*, pp. 379ff.
16. *Shabbat* 151b.
17. *Sepher Chassidim*, no. 724.
18. Ibid., no. 186.
19. Eleazar Fleckeles, responsa *Teshuvah Me'ahavah*, 1:53.
20. M. J. Zweig, in *No'am*, vol. 7, Jerusalem, p. 36 (1964).
21. *Hil. Rotze'ach*, 2:7.
22. Ibid.
23. Ibid., 8.
24. See Jakobovits, *Jewish Medical Ethics*, pp. 275ff.
25. Gen. 1:27; 5:1-3; cf. Deut. 21:23 and commentaries.
26. Gen. 30:1.
27. *Berachot* 5a.

28. See chapters "Law and Life" and "Law and Pain," in Jakobovits, *Jewish Medical Ethics*, pp. 45ff., and 99ff.

29. See "The Medical Treatment of Animals in Jewish Law," in Jakobovits, *The Timely and the Timeless*, pp. 368ff.

30. *Sanhedrin* 45a. See Jakobovits, *Jewish Medical Ethics*, p. 105. It should be added, however, that in practice Jewish law abolished the death penalty two thousand years ago or more, by making its imposition contingent on virtually impossible conditions, e.g., the evidence, and prior cautioning of the offender, by two eye-witnesses.

Eike-Henner W. Kluge

Infanticide as the Murder of Persons

1.

Infanticide has recently become the subject of increasing legal,[1] medical,[2] and philosophical attention,[3] and has been linked closely to discussions of abortion and euthanasia. For instance, it has been argued on purely moral grounds that since infants are not persons in any morally relevant sense, infanticide is really on a par with abortion and that, although both involve deliberate acts of killing, neither is an act of murder.[4] On purely medical grounds it has been suggested that infanticide is necessary to prevent a squandering of scarce medical resources which could be better employed helping those able to benefit from them, rather than being wasted on "seriously defective neonates" that will die sooner or later anyway.[5] Eugenic considerations have also been adduced,[6] as have been arguments stressing the burden imposed on family and society by the existence of children suffering from such debilities as spina bifida, thalidomide-induced morphological damage and abnormalities, Down's syndrome, etc.[7] Nor have all arguments focused on the benefits that would accrue to family and society were such infants to be killed: It has also been suggested that these children should be killed "for their own good,"[8] and that to keep them alive is to commit an injustice on their person.[9] It has even been proposed that recognition of the personhood of such infants should be withheld until an acceptable disposition concerning them has been made, so as to avoid legal complications.[10] Presumably, in the relevant cases, personhood would then be withheld entirely.

I intend to take a critical stance vis-à-vis most of these suggestions. That is to say, I intend to argue that almost without exception acts of infanticide are acts of murder; and murder not in some legalistic sense relative to a given point of law, but morally: as the deliberate and inexcusable killing of a person. My strategy in arguing this will be the following: I shall begin by defining 'infanticide', consider briefly the notion of personhood, and then give a definition of 'person'. I shall argue that it follows from this that infants are persons in a morally relevant sense. I shall then examine the notion of the right to life vis-à-vis the deontological presupposition-structure of rights, and from this go on to show that almost without exception, infanticide is murder. I shall conclude with a brief look at some possible objections to my train of reasoning.

2.

For the purpose of this discussion I shall understand the term 'infant' as it is defined in the legal context in which the problem of infanticide generally arises: a newborn child or neonate, a child within the first year of life. As to the concept of personhood, it is more difficult to adumbrate. Let me begin by distinguishing between it and that of a human being. The latter is an essentially biological concept denoting membership in the species *homo sapiens*. Its criteria of application are material in nature and involve such parameters as morphology, geneology or ancestry, genetic make-up and the like.[11] The concept of a person, on the other hand, involves notions like those of volition, perceptual awareness, desire, memory, expectation, the ability to reason and form judgments, self-awareness, etc. Therefore the two concepts are logically distinct—a fact that becomes all the more apparent when we note that the concept of a person also grounds the ascription of moral predicates, something that the biological concept of a human being does not and cannot do. Since it is this predicate-grounding feature of the notion of a person that is important in the present context, I shall henceforth ignore that of a human being and deal with that of a person alone.

Here, two questions immediately arise: How can personhood ground the ascription of moral predicates? and, What makes something a person? The first question belongs to pure, not applied, ethics. I shall therefore disregard it. As to the second, I have already given some intimation of what is involved: perceptual awareness, volition and desire, memory and expectation, the ability to reason and form judgments, self-awareness, and the like.[12] However, although to a greater or lesser degree all are involved in the concept of a person, not all are necessary constituents of it. Thus, while we should be inclined to call someone who has no desires, likes, or volitions inhuman, or someone without aesthetic sensibilities whatever a boor, we should not for all that refuse to call him a person. Similarly, while we should account someone without memories and expectations exceedingly peculiar, even psychologically deviant, his personhood would not be in question on this account, as the annals of psychiatry clearly illustrate. Only the following are really considered necessary for personhood: perceptual awareness, the ability to reason or form judgments, and self-awareness.

Of these, the first two are relatively unproblematic. Self-awareness, however, presents a difficulty. In the present context I can only say that it is not an item in consciousness but a manner of being aware: a mode of awareness that involves as one of its structuring moments a distinction between the individual as an entity within the universe, and the rest of the universe of which he is aware. As such, it also involves a body image. However, the latter need not be well defined or incorporate all of the modalities in which we are usually sensibly aware. As studies of postoperative traumas and of the development of infantile perceptual and motor skills have shown, it may increase in precision as well as undergo structural changes.

A person, then, is someone who is perceptually aware, has the ability to reason and form judgments, and is self-aware. However, as a definition, this is far too restrictive: It is couched in terms of actuality and hence rules out cases of what we unequivocally recognize to be persons but where not all of these criteria are actually present. Instances of deep coma, of anesthesia, here come to mind. Accordingly, the preceding characterization must be amended to include the potential for these characteristics. Not, of course, the potential in a pure and unqualified sense, but in the sense in which the actualization of this potential, were it to occur, would not require a constitutive structural change in the make-up of the entity involved. I shall call this a constitutive potential. The notion of a person can now be characterized like this:

> An entity is a person if and only if *either* it now is perceptually aware, reasons and makes judgments, and is self-aware, *or* it is in a state of constitutive potential with respect to these.

As to criteria of application, the first clause of this disjunction presents no difficulties; it is the second that poses a problem: How is the presence of such a constitutive potential to be determined? The answer lies in the fact that even in the paradigm case of a normal adult human being fulfilling the first clause, the actual presence of these defining characteristics is a function of the present physiological states of the individual in question: of the neurological activity of his brain.[13] This activity is associated with a particular type of EEG that, like the neurological activity that it indicates, is distinct from that of all other animals. Although normally we ascribe personhood on the basis of external behavioral manifestations, we could also go by the individual's neurological activity as indicated by his EEG. Therefore, the presence of an EEG structurally similar to that of a normal adult human being is sufficient to establish the actual presence of personhood, even if the normal and overt behavioral manifestations are wanting.

However, the matter goes deeper. The neurological activity of the brain, whether evidenced by overt external behavior or EEGs, is itself a function of the structure of the brain itself. Therefore by-passing all such criteria, we can appeal directly to the structure of the brain itself; and since the constitutive potential in the above sense is grounded in the present constitution of what has that potential and merely as it were awaits its actualization, this immediately provides the criterion necessary for determining whether the second clause of the preceding definition of 'person' is met:

> An entity has the constitutive potential for being perceptually aware, reasoning and making judgments, and for being self-aware if and only if its neurological system is structurally similar to that of a normal adult human being.[14]

3.

Given the definition of 'person' and the criteria for its application, I now turn to the question: At what point in the development of a human being are we faced with a person?

Clearly it is the first and not the second clause of the definition that is here germane; and the reply is that, generally speaking, by the end of the fourth month of the gestation period, certainly by the sixth, the constitutive potential for personhood is present. Differently, at that point the brain of the fetus is structurally and functionally sufficiently developed so as to leave no doubt that the above criteria for personhood in the constitutive sense are met. This is some time before actual birth. Consequently there is no question but that neonates also normally meet the requirements for personhood: that they are persons. Therefore, all other things being equal, to commit infanticide is to commit murder.

However, there is that phrase "all other things being equal." It suggests that things are not always equal: that, whereas infants normally are persons and do have the rights of persons, they do not always have them, or do not have them in the same degree—that such rights are defeasible—and that therefore in their case there are exceptive and/or excusing conditions that ameliorate what otherwise would be a charge of murder. Certain recent arguments raise precisely this sort of consideration, and the following two may be taken as representative: (1) Since neonates have no concept of life, they lack the desire to live and therefore do not have any right to life.[15] (2) The neonates' lack of full social interaction and role entails that, whereas they do have such rights as that to freedom from torture, they do not have the right to life.[16] In either case, therefore, to commit infanticide is not to commit murder.

Consistency demands that the preceding cannot be the import of the qualifying clause in my previous assertion. However, before clarifying what the latter does amount to, I should like to deal briefly with the two arguments just indicated, since they are of some theoretical importance. To begin with the first: The thesis on which it is based is the general claim that someone has a right to R if and only if he has the concept of R and desires R. But why should anyone accept this claim? Not only is it counterintuitive, it also contradicts ordinary practice. Animals are said to have rights, e.g., to freedom from torture, and neonates likewise, yet neither has the relevant concept. Neonates also are said to have the right to freedom from slavery, yet this concept can hardly be claimed as part of their intellectual accoutrement. Examples could be multiplied. Furthermore, there is this fundamental question: Why should the existence of a conceptualized desire in itself be the basis of a right?[17] If it were, then a murderer would have a prima facie right to the death of his victim, a thief to the goods of his fellow man, and a dictator to world domination. In actuality, of course, it is not the desires, conceptualized or otherwise, that ground the rights but the nature and status of the individual himself; and once an entity is a person, all the rights that depend on personhood belong to him. Of course this does not mean that all rights are grounded in personhood. Some require certain types of actions, social interrelations, etc. The right to life, however, is not of this sort.

As to the second objection—that an infant may have the right to freedom from torture and sundry other rights but lack the right to life—this bespeaks a confusion over the deontological interrelationship among rights. Rights have what could be called a presuppositional structure. That is to say, the existence of a right trivially entails the right to exercise it. This in turn entails that if certain conditions are necessary for the exercise of that right, then the individual also has the right to bring these about. Therefore someone can have right R only if he also has rights P and O, the exercise of which is a necessary precondition for the exercise of R. Now the objection itself grants that infants have rights, e.g., the right to freedom from torture. That right, however, as indeed any other right, presupposes the existence of whatever has it—in this case, of the infant. Therefore, the infant also has the right to life.[18]

However, this reply in terms of the presupposition–structure of rights itself raises two questions: (1) Does this not entail that, since animals also have rights such as that to freedom from torture, they too have a right to life? Indeed, as much as do persons? (2) What of situations involving conflicts of rights? For instance, the existence of an infant may threaten not merely the emotional, social, and physical well-being of its family but, considered from a holistic point of view, the very existence of the society into which it is born. After all, there is only a finite amount of resources. Consequently, is it not reasonable that under such conditions purely utilitarian considerations prevail? All the more so since if they do not, the infant is likely to end as a statistic of the battered child syndrome?

The answer to (1) is that the presupposition-structure of rights does indeed entail that animals have a right to life. But it does not entail that this right is indefeasible—particularly when it conflicts with the rights of persons. In other words, rights can be ranked not only with respect to their natures but also with respect to whose rights they are. Consequently, a right had by one individual may not be effective in face of the very same right had by another individual of a different nature. The rights of persons and animals, therefore, even when they are the same, are not the same.

As to (2), it seeks to create the impression that the sort of situation it envisages constitutes a conflict matrix that can be resolved only by the subjugation of the right to life of the infant. That, however, is erroneous. The key to understanding why lies in realizing that moral agents are responsible for the normally foreseeable effects of their actions. In procreating under the above circumstances, the participants to that act have assumed responsibility for the existence of a new living being, the fetus, and have subordinated their rights to its rights[19]—commensurate, of course, with the degree of development of the fetus involved.[20] In itself, this does not entail that in situations of conflicting rights to life, etc., the conflict must always be resolved in favor of the fetus. The reply to (1) above should have made this clear. However, in permitting the fetus to develop until it has attained personhood, the parents (and society) have assumed responsibility for the existence not merely of a living being but of a person, and have *de facto* confirmed the subordination of the normal exercise of their rights *even in the sphere of life and death* to that of the new person. Therefore, the right to life of the infant normally does take precedence,[21] and when a conflict of rights obtains, it must be normally resolved in favor of the infant.

Of course the conflict matrix as set out in (2) is unnecessarily restrictive. Rarely is the situation as desperate as (2) makes out. Generally the problem—or the likelihood of such a problem—can be averted by a restructuring of social institutions to reflect the fact that the advent of a new person is not only a familial but also a social responsibility. Such a restructuring may and perhaps ought to include laws governing who may have children, when, under what circumstances, and what role society should play in their support. Of course, if despite all this the conditions should become as desperate as (2) makes out, then, consonant with the deontological relationship among rights indicated, the rights of those directly responsible for the existence of the new person must take a subordinate place. It goes almost without saying that the attempt to justify infanticide as a means of avoiding an increase in the number of victims of the battered child syndrome is morally unacceptable. Morally, the situation calls for what I have just indicated: a recognition of the social as well as familial responsibility for neonates, and the implementation of appropriate social institutions.

4.

I now turn to the qualifying conditions governing infanticide that I mentioned a few paragraphs ago. In raising the issue at all, I suggested that the right to life of an infant is not indefeasible: that it is not always effective. I should now like to clarify how this is to be understood, and how I could propose such conditions without doing violence to the logic of my position. In order to do so, and at the same time to provide some insight into the actual operation of the thesis that I have sketched, I shall deal with it in the context of some objections that could be raised against what I have argued.

(a)

[In the case of seriously defective neonates] life-preserving intervention must be understood as doing harm to an individual who cannot survive infancy, or who will be in intolerable pain, or cannot participate even minimally in human experience.[22]

This objection seeks to justify infanticide by admitting the personhood of infants and therefore their right to life, but at the same time suggesting that the interrelationship among rights is not as I have sketched; that the right to freedom from intolerable pain or subnormal human experience takes precedence over the right to life:[23] that in some cases the quality of life is a weightier consideration than the life itself. Therefore in some cases, particularly those mentioned, infanticide is morally called for.[24]

Let me agree at the outset that in some instances to keep someone alive is to infringe on his rights as a person. However, as an objection to what I have argued, this fails. It confuses the ranking of rights—their presupposition-structure—with their weight. The former involves the deontological conditions under which someone has a right; the latter concerns the conditions under which he may choose to exercise it. Which rights are exercised is a function of their weight in a given context, not of their presupposition-structure. Therefore, while the right to life is indeed presupposed by the right to freedom from intolerable pain, this does not entail that in all contexts the former is more effective than the latter. Furthermore, the objection also ignores the fact that under certain circumstances a right can be exercised by someone for someone else—for instance, when an immediate decision about the physiological disposition of an individual must be made, e.g., rè an operation, but the person himself is incapacitated. Here others may and indeed must exercise the right of choice for the individual; and if the decision is based on the best data available under the circumstances, the prognosis is as indicated, and the choice is one that a reasonable person would have made, then it is as though the individual himself had made it, and we are right to act on it. The situation of "seriously defective neonates" must be considered in this light, and under the sorts of circumstances outlined in the objection the decision may well be for death.[25] But it need not be. It all depends. Infanticide, therefore, need not be murder. However, it is important to note why this is so: not because there are exceptive clauses for certain kinds of infanticide as such, but because certain putative cases of infanticide are in fact not cases of infanticide at all but of agent suicide.

(b)

In cases of limited availability of neonatal intensive care, it is ethical to terminate therapy for an infant with poor prognosis in order to provide care for an infant with much better prognosis.[26]

To be morally persuasive, the position here indicated must be understood as to the effect that the giving of intensive care to a neonate with poor prognosis results in the unavailability of such care to one with "much better prognosis," that with such care the latter will (probably) survive, but that if it were shared, both neonates will (probably) die.

The suggestion here is that acceptance of what I have argued entails the last (eminently counterintuitive) decision, that therefore I am wrong, and that in this sort of case infanticide is morally acceptable. However, the objection misses the mark. Once more, what we have here is not a properly and uniquely infanticidal situation involving a question about the personhood of infants or the nature and relationship of their rights vis-à-vis ours. Instead, it is a special version of the general problem of the allocation of limited medical—indeed, of any life-giving and sustaining —resources when these cannot be distributed to all without ensuring the death of all but which, if given to a select few, will guarantee their survival. In short, it is a problem of *triage*. And the solution is that in such bipolar contexts where there is no gradation of effects, pragmatic considerations become decisive. In other words, the preceding is an instance of a conflict-of-rights problem among persons, not of infanticide as such; and the solution here must be the same as in all other *triage* situations involving persons. It has no special significance for my thesis.

(c)

It is argued that a mongoloid or otherwise seriously defective infant should be killed or left to die: for the good of the infant, for the sake of avoiding difficulties for the family, and for the good of society.[27]

Once again, however, this does not militate against my position. If the mental deficiency of the neonate is so great as to disqualify it from personhood, then killing it will not be murder; if it does not disqualify it, then prima facie to kill it will be to commit murder. Any claim to the contrary will have to establish, on the basis of independent argument, the moral correctness of the utilitarian considerations underlying the objection—or, alternately, show that we are here faced with a conflict-of-rights situation where the infant must lose. The claim that it will be for the good of the infant can be dismissed on factual grounds: almost invariably such mentally defective neonates are happy individuals.[28] Furthermore, this objection seems to equate personhood with the possession of a certain level of intelligence. Although the two are indeed connected in that a certain minimal degree of intelligence is necessary for self-awareness and perceptual awareness of reality, etc., this does not entail the portmanteau denial of personhood to all mentally defective neonates. It all depends on whether the criteria for personhood are met in the particular case. We must look and see. If they are met, even if only minimally, then to procure death will be to commit murder.

(d)

It is argued that there should be a social policy that [withholds] legal personhood from certain carefully defined categories of high risk infants until a clear diagnosis and prognosis can be made concerning them.[29]

This line of argumentation fails because it construes personhood as a legal convention that can be given or withheld, depending on the pragmatics of the situation. Legally, this may be the case; morally it is not, as viz., the first part of my discussion. The personhood of an individual is not a function of any conventions that we choose to apply or refrain from applying, but instead is a status that depends on whether or not the individual meets certain factual criteria. Therefore while to withhold personhood might possibly solve certain legal problems—but precisely how are these "categories" to be defined without including or excluding too much?—this would simply ignore the moral ones. In other words, this objection amounts to a confusion of legal with moral personhood.

(e)
An infant should be killed in cases of severe physiological debility, such as spina bifida, where prognosis is for a short and abnormal life.[30]

Two points are here important: one, that this particular position does not deny the personhood of the infants; and two, that if it is to be understood differently from (a) and (c), then it must be construed as a pragmatic appeal to the burden imposed on parents and society by the existence of such infants. In that case, however, it reduces to the thesis that when the inconvenience and cost engendered by an infant's existence exceed or threaten to exceed a certain maximum without an adequate degree of return, then either he no longer has a right to life, or that right is superseded by the right to convenience, etc., on the part of parents and society. However, since the personhood of these infants is not in question, this in turn must be seen as a particular version of a general thesis dealing with the rights of persons as such when their existence becomes too burdensome or inconvenient for family and society: When the inconvenience and cost engendered for family and society by the existence of a *person* exceed or threaten to exceed a certain maximum without adequate return, then either that person no longer has a right to life, or that right is superseded by the right to convenience, etc., on the part of family and society. In other words, it will be morally all right to kill such a person.

Unless my analysis is wholly mistaken, the general thesis amounts to permission to murder for the sake of convenience, and the counsel for infanticide is but a particular version of this. However, the general thesis, its particular version, and the utilitarianism that underlies it require detailed and independent argument, especially vis-à-vis what I have said about the ranking of rights and persons. As it stands, it is merely an unacceptable and unargued counterclaim.

Cases and analyses could be multiplied, but the preceding affords some insight into what is entailed by the personhood that, if I am correct, belongs to most infants. In particular it shows that most infants are persons, and that unless their right to life is superseded by the rights of other persons, as in (b), or their status as persons and particular situation combine to require euthanasia, as in (a), to kill them is to commit murder.

By way of summing up, let me return to the title of this paper: It is a pleonasm, and deliberately so in order to focus on the fact that, by and large, infanticide is murder, and that this is a direct consequence of the status of infants as persons. I should be naive if I thought that in giving this moral analysis of infanticide I had solved the social and economic problems that frequently underlie the killing of "seriously defective neonates." I can only hope for a speedy realization of society's responsibility towards infants as persons—for instance, by means of adequate legislation in the social and medical sphere—so that the pragmatic pressures to effect a livable solution for the family will no longer lead to murder.

Notes

1. E.g., Glanville Williams, *The Sanctity of Life and the Criminal Law* (Salem, N.H.: Faber and Faber, 1958); J. A. Robertson, "Involuntary Euthanasia of Defective Newborns: A Legal Analysis," *Stanford Law Review* 27 (January 1975): 213-67; J. Sanders, "Euthanasia. None Dare Call It Murder," *Journal of Criminal Law, Criminology and Police Science* 60 (1969): 97-107.

2. E.g., Report of the 65th Ross Conference on Pediatric Research: *Ethical Dilemmas in Current Obstetric and Newborn Care* (Columbus: Ross Laboratories, 1973); Diana Crane, *The Sanctity of Social Life: Physicians' Treatment of the Critically Ill* (New York: Russell Sage Foundation, 1975); Richard Trubo, *An Act of Mercy: Euthanasia Today* (Los Angeles: Nash Publishing, 1973); Earl R. Babbie, *Science and Morality in Medicine: A Survey of Medical Educators* (Berkeley, Calif.: University of California Press, 1970); A. R. Jonsen, R. H. Phibbs, W. W. Tooley, and M. J. Garlan, "Critical Issues in Newborn Intensive Care: A Conference Report and Policy Proposal," *Journal of the American Medical Association* 55, no. 6 (June 1975): 756-68; R. S. Duff and A. G. M. Campbell, "Moral and Ethical Dilemmas in the Special Care Nursery," *New England Journal of Medicine* 289 (1973): 890; J. Lorber, "Criteria of Selection of Patients for Treatment," *Proceedings of the Fourth International Conference on Birth Defects (Vienna, 1973);* J. Freeman, "To Treat or Not to Treat: Ethical Dilemmas of Treating the Infant with Myelomeningocele," *Clinical Neurosurgery* 20 (1973): 134; H. T. Engelhardt, Jr., "Euthanasia and Children: The Injury of Continued Existence," *Journal of Pediatrics* 83 (1973): 170—to mention but a few.

3. Cf. Michael Tooley, "A Defense of Abortion and Infanticide," in *The Problem of Abortion,* ed. Joel Feinberg (Belmont, Calif.: Wadsworth, 1973), pp. 51-91; S. I. Benn, "Abortion, Infanticide and Respect for Persons," in *Problem of Abortion,* pp. 92-104; E.-H. W. Kluge, *The Practice of Death* (New Haven, Conn.: Yale University Press, 1975); Robert Veatch, *Death, Dying and the Biological Revolution* (New Haven, Conn.: Yale University Press, 1976), especially pp. 123-154; Marvin Kohl, *The Morality of Killing* (New York: Humanities Press and London: Peter Owen, 1974); etc.

4. See especially Tooley, "Defense of Abortion and Infanticide," and Benn, "Abortion, Infanticide and Respect," both in Feinberg, *Problem of Abortion.*

5. Cf. Jonsen et al., "Issues in Newborn Intensive Care," pp. 761-63, especially p. 763.

6. Cf. Williams, *Sanctity of Life,* pp. 18ff.

7. Cf. R. B. Zachary, "Ethical and Social Aspects of Treatment of Spina Bifida," *Lancet* 2 (1968): 274-76; R. C. Sanders, "Spina Bifida: A Reply to R. B. Zachary," *Lancet* 2 (1968): 457; J. M. Gustafson, "Mongolism, Parental Desire and the Right to Life," *Perspectives in Biology and Medicine* 16 (1973): 529, especially pp. 544-45. Gustafson opposes this reasoning.

8. Cf. Gustafson, "Mongolism, Parental Desire and Right to Life."

9. Jonsen et al., "Issues in Newborn Intensive Care," p. 760; and Engelhardt, "Euthanasia and Children."

10. Jonsen et al., "Issues in Newborn Intensive Care," p. 758.

11. Cf. Kluge, *Practice of Death,* pp. 88ff.

12. Cf. Tooley, "Defense of Abortion," in Feinberg, *Problem of Abortion,* pp. 63, 72, passim; Trubo, *Act of Mercy,* p. 152; etc.

13. Cf. Kluge, *Practice of Death,* pp. 91-95; Tooley, "Defense of Abortion," in Feinberg, *Problem of Abortion,* p. 77.

14. This criterion also has the not inconsiderable advantage of allowing the above definition of 'person' to apply to unusual cases, such as that of a comatose individual with a silver plate in his skull who does not ever give normal EEGs.

15. Cf. Tooley, "Defense of Abortion," in Feinberg, *Problem of Abortion,* pp. 69ff., 91, etc.; Benn, "Abortion, Infanticide and Respect," in Feinberg, *Problem of Abortion,* p. 99; Trubo, *Act of Mercy,* p. 152, etc.

16. Cf. Tooley, "Defense of Abortion," in Feinberg, *Problem of Abortion.*

17. It will be apparent why nothing else will do: An instinctive desire would obviate an argument such as Tooley's, "Defense of Abortion," or Benn's, "Abortion, Infanticide and Respect," in Feinberg, *Problem of Abortion,* p. 99.

18. Of course, it could be argued that rights in general and the right to life in particular really are conditional on the possession of certain attributes, as suggested above, and therefore would be expressed more correctly like this:

'A has the right to life' means 'If A exists and is a person, then A has a right to life' (Cf. Tooley, "Defense of Abortion," in Feinberg, *Problem of Abortion,* p. 69).

However, since it is clear from the preceding that the conditions of the antecedent are met, the consequent follows. The only way to avoid this is to make the right to life conditional not on the possession of personhood but some other characteristic. That, however, would have to be argued. Prima facie it is not clear how such an argument would proceed without running into conflict with the presupposition-structure of rights sketched above.

19. Incidentally, this also includes the society that permits the act.

20. Obviously, this precludes treating the fetus at any stage as mere tissue, as has been suggested in some medical circles. (Cf. Paul Ramsey, *The Ethics of Fetal Research*[New Haven, Conn.: Yale University Press, 1975] who opposes this.) Minimally, their moral status is equivalent to that of a neurologically correspondingly developed animal.

21. For exceptive circumstances, see below.

22. Jonsen et. al., "Issues in Newborn Intensive Care," p. 760; cf. Sanders, "Euthanasia."

23. Cf. Tooley, "Defense of Abortion," in Feinberg, *Problem of Abortion.* I ignore the essentially pragmatic aspects of survival beyond infancy and deal with it below.

24. Cf. Kluge, *Practice of Death,* chap. IV; I consider subhuman mental existence below.

25. Whether death is to be engendered actively or passively is irrelevant. Cf. Kluge, *Practice of Death,* p. 156, n. 20; Veatch, *Death, Dying and the Biological Revolution,* pp. 77-104.

26. Jonsen et al., "Issues of Newborn Intensive Care," p. 761; cf. Crane, *Sanctity of Social Life,* p. 133, also pp. 213-267; Trubo, *Act of Mercy,* p. 153.

27. Gustafson, "Mongolism, Parental Desire and the Right to Life," pp. 544-45; Trubo, *Act of Mercy*, pp. 142ff.

28. Gustafson, "Mongolism, Parental Desire and the Right to Life," passim.

29. Jonsen et al., "Issues in Newborn Intensive Care," p. 758.

30. Cf. Sanders, "Euthanasia"; G. K. Smith and E. D. Smith, "Selection for Treatment in Spina Bifida Cystica," *Brit. Med. Jour.* 4 (1973): 189; S. C. Stein, L. Schut, and M. D. Ames, "Selection for Early Treatment in Myelomeningocele: A Retrospective Analysis of Various Selection Procedures," *M.A.M.A.* 55, no. 5 (November 1974): 553-57; etc.

Richard B. Brandt

Defective Newborns and the Morality of Termination

The *legal* rights of a fetus are very different from those of a newborn. The fetus may be aborted, legally, for any reason or no reason up to twenty-four or twenty-eight weeks (U.S. Supreme Court, *Roe* v. *Wade*). But, at least in theory, immediately after birth an infant has all the legal rights of the adult, including the right to life.

The topic of this paper, however, is to identify the moral rights of the newborn, specifically whether *defective* newborns have a right to life. But it is simpler to talk, not about "rights to life," but about when or whether it is *morally right* either actively or passively (by withdrawal of life-supportive measures) to terminate defective newborns. It is also better because the conception of a right involves the notion of a sphere of autonomy—something is to be done or omitted, but only if the subject of the rights wants or consents—and this fact is apt to be confusing or oversimplifying. Surely what we want to know is whether termination is morally right or wrong, and nothing can turn on the semantics of the concept of a "right."[1]

What does one have to do in order to support some answer to these questions? One thing we can do is ask—and I think myself that the answer to this question is definitive for our purposes—whether rational or fully informed persons would, in view of the total consequences, support a moral code for a society in which they expected to live, with one, or another, provision on this matter. (I believe a fully rational person will at least normally have some degree of benevolence, or positive interest in the welfare or happiness of others; I shall not attempt to specify how much.) Since, however, I do not expect that everyone else will agree that answering this question would show what is morally right, I shall, for their benefit, also argue that certain moral principles on this matter are coherent with strong moral convictions of reflective people; or, to use Rawls's terminology, that a certain principle on the matter would belong to a system of moral principles in "reflective equilibrium."

Historically, many writers, including Pope Pius XI in *Casti Connubii* (1930), have affirmed an absolute prohibition against killing anyone who is neither guilty of a capital crime nor an unjust assailant threatening one's life (self-defense), except in case of "extreme necessity." Presumably the prohibition is intended to include withholding of food or liquid from a newborn, although strictly speaking this is only *failing* to do something, not actually *doing* something to bring about a death. (Would writers in this tradition demand, on moral grounds, that complicated and expensive surgery be undertaken to save a life? Such surgery is going beyond normal care, and in some cases beyond what earlier writers even conceived.) However the intentions of these writers may be, we should observe that historically their moral condemnation of all killing (except for the cases mentioned) derives from the Biblical injunction, "Thou shalt not kill," which, as it stands and without interpretation, may be taken to forbid suicide, killing of animals, perhaps even plants, and hence cannot be taken seriously.

Presumably a moral code that is coherent with our intuitions and that rational persons would support for their society would include some prohibition of killing, but it is another matter to identify the exact class to which such a prohibition is to apply. For one thing, I would doubt that killing one's self would be included—although one might be forbidden to kill one's self if that would work severe hardship on others, or conflict with the discharge of one's other moral obligations. And, possibly, defective newborns would *not* be included in the class. Further, a decision has to be made whether the prohibition of killing is *absolute* or only *prima facie*, meaning by "prima facie" that the duty not to kill might be outweighed by some other duty (or right) stronger in the circumstances, which could be fulfilled only by killing. In case this distinction is made, we would have to decide whether defective newborns fall within the scope of even a prima facie moral prohibition against killing. I shall, however, not attempt to make this fine distinction here, and shall simply inquire whether, everything considered, defective newborns—or some identifiable group of them—are excluded from the moral prohibition against killing.

THE PROSPECTIVE QUALITY OF LIFE
OF DEFECTIVE NEWBORNS

Suppose that killing a defective newborn, or allowing it to die, would not be an *injury*, but would rather be doing the infant a favor. In that case we should feel intuitively less opposed to termination of newborns, and presumably rational persons would be less inclined to support a moral code with a prohibition against such action. In that case we would feel rather as we do about a person's preventing a suicide attempt from being successful, in order that the person be elaborately tortured to death at a later stage. It is no favor to the prospective suicide to save his life; similarly, if the prospective life of defective newborns is bad we are doing them a favor to let them die.

It may be said that we have no way of knowing what the conscious experiences of defective children are like, and that we have no competence in any case to decide when or what kind of life is bad or not worth living. Further, it may be said that predictions about a defective newborn's prospects for the future are precarious, in view of possible further advances of medicine. It does seem, however, that here, as everywhere, the rational person will follow the evidence about the present or future facts. But there is a question how to decide whether a life is bad or not worth living.

In the case of *some* defective newborns, it seems clear that their prospective life is bad. Suppose, as sometimes happens, a child is hydrocephalic with an extremely low I.Q., is blind and deaf, has no control over its body, can only lie on its back all day and have all its needs taken care of by others, and even cries out with pain when it is touched or lifted. Infants born with spina bifida—and these number over two per one thousand births—are normally not quite so badly off, but are often nearly so.

But what criterion are we using if we say that such a life is bad? One criterion might be called a "happiness" criterion. If a person *likes* a moment of experience while he is having it, his life is so far good; if a person *dislikes* a moment of experience while he is having it, his life is so far bad. Based on such reactions, we might construct a "happiness curve" for a person, going up above the indifference axis when a moment of experience is liked—and how far above depending on how strongly it is liked—and dipping down below the line when a moment is disliked. Then this criterion would say that a life is worth living if there is a net balance of positive area under the curve over a lifetime, and that it is bad if there is a net balance of negative area. One might adopt some different criterion: for instance, one might say that a life is worth living if a person would *want* to live it over again given that, at the end, he could remember the whole of it with perfect vividness in some kind of grand intuitive awareness. Such a response to this hypothetical holistic intuition, however, would likely be affected by the state of the person's drives or moods at the time, and the conception strikes me as unconvincing, compared with the moment-by-moment reaction to what is going on. Let us, for the sake of the argument, adopt the happiness criterion.[2]

Is the prospective life of the seriously defective newborn, like the one described above, bad or good according to this criterion? One thing seems clear: that it is *less* good than is the prospective life of a normal infant. But is it bad?

We have to do some extrapolating from what we know. For instance, such a child will presumably suffer from severe sensory deprivation; he is simply not getting interesting stimuli. On the basis of laboratory data, it is plausible to think the child's experience is at best boring or uncomfortable. If the child's experience is painful, of course, its moments are, so far, on the negative side. One must suppose that such a child hardly suffers from disappointment, since it will not learn to expect anything exciting, beyond being fed and fondled, and these events will be regularly forthcoming. One might expect such a child to suffer from isolation and loneliness, but insofar as this is true, the object of dislike probably should be classified as just sensory deprivation; dislike of loneliness seems to depend on the deprivation of past pleasures of human company. There are also some positive enjoyments: of eating, drinking, elimination, seeing the nurse coming with food, and so on. But the brief enjoyments can hardly balance the long stretches of boredom, discomfort, or even pain. On the whole, the lives of such children are bad according to the happiness criterion.

Naturally we cannot generalize about the cases of all "defective"

RICHARD B. BRANDT

newborns; there are all sorts of defects, and the cases I have described are about the worst. A child with spina bifida may, if he survives the numerous operations, I suppose, adjust to the frustrations of immobility; he may become accustomed to the embarrassments of no bladder or bowel control; he may have some intellectual enjoyments like playing chess; he will suffer from observing what others have but he cannot, such as sexual satisfactions, in addition to the pain of repeated surgery. How does it all balance out? Surely not as very good, but perhaps above the indifference level.

It may fairly be said, I think, that the lives of some defective newborns are destined to be bad on the whole, and it would be a favor to them if their lives were terminated. Contrariwise, the prospective lives of many defective newborns are modestly pleasant, and it would be some injury to them to be terminated, albeit the lives they will live are ones some of us would prefer not to live at all.

CONSENT

Let us now make a second suggestion, not this time that termination of a defective newborn would be doing him a favor, but this time that he *consents* to termination, in the sense of expressing a rational deliberated preference for this. In that case I suggest that intuitively we would be *more* favorably inclined to judge that it is right to let the defective die, and I suggest also that for that case rational persons would be more ready to support a moral code permitting termination. Notice that we think that if an ill person has signified what we think a rational and deliberated desire to die, we are morally better justified in withdrawing life-supporting measures than we otherwise would be.

The newborn, however, is incapable of expressing his preference (giving consent) at all, much less expressing a rational deliberated preference. There could in theory be court-appointed guardians or proxies, presumably disinterested parties, authorized to give such consent on his behalf; but even so this would not be *his* consent.

Nevertheless, there is a fact about the mental life of the newborn (defective or not) such that, if he could understand the fact, it seems he would not object—even rationally or after deliberation, if that were possible—to his life being terminated, or to his parents substituting another

50

child in his place. This suggestion may seem absurd, but let us see. The explanation runs along the lines of an argument I once used to support the morality of abortion. I quote the paragraph in which this argument was introduced:[3]

> Suppose I were seriously ill, and were told that, for a sizeable fee, an operation to save "my life" could be performed, of the following sort: my brain would be removed to another body which could provide a normal life, but the unfortunate result of the operation would be that my memory and learned abilities would be wholly erased, and that the forming of memory brain traces must begin again from scratch, as in a newborn baby. Now, how large a fee would I be willing to pay for this operation, when the alternative is my peaceful demise? My own answer would be: None at all. I would take no interest in the continued existence of "myself" in that sense, and I would rather add the sizeable fee to the inheritance of my children. . . . I cannot see the point of forfeiting my children's inheritance in order to start off a person who is brand new except that he happens to enjoy the benefit of having my present brain, without the memory traces. It appears that some continuity of memory is a necessary condition for personal identity *in an important sense.*

My argument was that the position of a fetus, at the end of the first trimester, is essentially the same as that of the person contemplating this operation: he will consider that the baby born after six more months will not be *he* in any *important* and *motivating* sense (there will be no continuity of memory, and, indeed, maybe nothing to have been remembered), and the later existence of this baby, in a sense bodily continuous with his present body, would be a matter of indifference to him. So, I argued, nothing is being done to the fetus that he would object to having done if he understood the situation.

What do I think is necessary in order for the continuation of my body with its conscious experiences to be worthwhile? One thing is that it is able to remember the events I can now remember; another is that it takes some interest in the projects I am now planning and remembers them as my projects; another is that it recognizes my friends and has warm feelings for them, and so on. Reflection on these states of a future continuation of my body with its experiences is what makes the idea motivating. But such motivating reflection for a newborn is impossible: he has no memories that he wants recalled later; he has no plans to execute; he has no warm feelings for other persons. He has simply not had the length of life necessary for these to come about. Not only that: the conception of these things cannot be motivating because the concept of some state of affairs being motivating requires roughly a past experience in which similar states of affairs were satisfying, and he has not lived long enough for the requisite conditioning to have taken place. (The most one could say is that the image of warm milk in his mouth is attractive; he might answer affirmatively if it could be put to him whether he would be aversive to the idea of no more warm milk.) So we can say, not merely that the newborn does not want the continuation of himself as a subject of experiences (he has not the conceptual framework for this); he does not want *anything* that his own survival would promote. It is like the case of the operation: there is nothing I want that the survival of my brain with no memory would promote. Give the newborn as much *conceptual* framework as you like; the *wants* are not there, which could give significance to the continuance of his life.

The newborn, then, is bound to be *indifferent* to the idea of a continuation of the stream of his experiences, even if he clearly has the idea of that. It seems we can *know* this about him.

The truth of all this is still not for it to be the case that the newborn, defective or not, gives *consent* to, or expresses a preference for, the termination of his life. *Consent* is a performance, normally linguistic, but always requiring some conventional *sign*. A newborn, who has not yet learned how to signalize consent, cannot give consent. And it may be thought that this difference makes all the difference.

In order to see what difference it does make in this case, we should ask what makes adult consent morally important. Why is it that we think euthanasia can be practiced on an adult only if he gives his consent, at least his implied consent (e.g., by previous statements)? There seem to be two reasons. The first is that a person is more likely to be concerned with his own welfare, and to take steps to secure it, than are others, even his good friends. Giving an individual control over his own life, and not permitting others to take control except when he consents, is normally to promote his welfare. An individual may, of course, behave stupidly or shortsightedly, but we think that on the whole a person's welfare is best secured if decisions about it are in his hands; and it is best for society in the normal case (not for criminals, etc.) if persons' own lives are well-served. The second reason is the feeling of security a person can have, if he knows the major decisions about himself are in his own hands. When they are not, a person can easily, and in some cases very reasonably, suppose that other persons may well be able to do something to him that he would very much like them not to do. He does not have to worry about that if he knows they cannot do it without his consent.

Are things different with the newborn? At least he, like the fetus, is not yet able to suffer from insecurity; he cannot worry about what others may do to him. So the second reason for requiring consent cannot have any importance in his case. His situation is thus very unlike that of the senile adult, for an adult can worry about what others may do to him if they judge him senile. And this worry can well cast a shadow over a lot of life. But how about the first reason? Here matters are more complex. In the case of children, we think their own lives are better cared for if certain decisions are in the hands of others: the child may not want to visit the dentist, but the parents know that his best interests are served by going, and they make him go. The same for compulsory school attendance. And the same for the newborn. But there is another point: that society has an interest, at certain crucial points, that may not be served by doing just exactly what is for the lifelong interest of the newborn. There are huge costs that are relevant, in the case of the defective newborn. I shall go into that problem in a moment. It seems, then, that in the case of the newborn, *consent* cannot have the moral importance that it has in the case of adults.

On the other hand, then, the newborn will not *care* whether his life is terminated, even if he understands his situation perfectly; and, on the other hand, consent does not have the moral importance in his case that it has for adults. So, while it seems true that we would feel better about permitting termination of defective newborns if only they could give rational and deliberated consent and gave it, nevertheless when we bear the foregoing two points in mind, the absence of consent does not seem morally crucial in their case. We can understand why rational persons deciding which moral code to support for their society would not make the giving of consent a necessary condition for feeling free to terminate an infant's life when such action was morally indicated by the other features of the situation.

REPLACEMENT IN ORDER TO GET A BETTER LIFE

Let us now think of an example owing to Derek Parfit. Suppose a woman wants a child, but is told that if she conceives a child now it will be defective, whereas if she waits three months she will produce a normal child. Obviously we think it would be wrong for the mother not to delay. (If she delays, the child she will have is not the *same* child as the one she would have had if she had not delayed, but it will have a better life.) This is the sole reason why we think she should delay and have the later-born child.

Suppose, however, a woman conceives but discovers only three months later that the fetus will become a defective child, but that she can have a normal child if she has an abortion and tries again. Now this time there is still the same reason for having the abortion that there formerly was for the delay: that she will produce a child with a better life. Ought she not then to have the abortion? If the child's life is bad, he could well complain that he had been injured by deliberately being brought to term. Would he complain if he were aborted, in favor of the later normal child? Not if the argument of the preceding section is correct.

But now suppose the woman does not discover until after she gives birth, that the child is seriously defective, but that she could conceive again and have a normal child. Are things really different, in the first few days? One might think that a benevolent person would want, in each of these cases, the substitution of a normal child for the defective one, of the better life for the worse one.

THE COST AND ITS RELEVANCE

It is agreed that the burden of care for a defective infant, say one born with spina bifida, is huge. The cost of surgery alone for an infant with spina bifida has been estimated to be around $275,000.[4] In many places this cost must be met by the family of the child, and there is the additional cost of care in an institution, if the child's condition does not permit care at home—and a very modest estimate of the monthly cost at present is $1,100. To meet even the surgical costs, not to mention monthly payments for continuing care, the lives of members of the family must be at a most spartan level for many years. The psychological effects of this, and equally, if not more so, of care provided at home, are far-reaching; they are apt to destroy the marriage and to cause psychological problems for the siblings. There is the on-going anxiety, the regular visits, the continuing presence of a caretaker if the child is in the home. In one way or another the continued existence of the child is apt to reduce dramatically the quality of life of the family as a whole.

It can be and has been argued that such costs, while real, are irrelevant to the moral problem of what should be done.[5] It is obvious, however, that rational persons, when deciding which moral code to support, would take these human costs into account. As indeed they should: the parents and siblings are also human beings with lives to live, and any sacrifices a given law or moral system might call on them to make must be taken into account in deciding between laws and moral codes. Everyone will feel sympathy for a helpless newborn; but everyone should also think, equally vividly, of all the others who will suffer and just how they will suffer—and, of course, as indicated above, of just what kind of life the defective newborn will have in any case. There is a choice here between allowing a newborn to die (possibly a favor to it, and in any case not a serious loss), and imposing a very heavy burden on the family for many years to come.

Philosophers who think the cost to others is irrelevant to what should be done should reflect that we do not accept the general principle that lives should be saved at no matter what cost. For instance, ships are deliberately built with only a certain margin of safety; they could be built so that they would hardly sink in any storm, but to do so would be economically unfeasible. We do not think we should require a standard of safety for automobiles that goes beyond a certain point of expense and inconvenience; we are prepared to risk a few extra deaths. And how about the lives we are willing to lose in war, in order to assure a certain kind of economic order or democracy or free speech? Surely there is a point at which the loss of a life (or the abbreviation of a life) and the cost to others become comparable. Is it obvious that the continuation of a marginal kind of life for a child takes moral precedence over providing a college education for one or more of his siblings? Some comparisons will be hard to make, but continuing even a marginally pleasant life hardly has absolute priority.

DRAWING LINES

There are two questions which must be answered in any complete account of what is the morally right thing to do about defective newborns.

The first is: If a decision to terminate is made, how soon must it be made? Obviously it could not be postponed to the age of five, or of three, or even a year and a half. At those ages, all the reasons for insisting on consent are already cogent. And at those ages, the child will already care what happens to him. But ten days is tolerable. Doubtless advances in medicine will permit detection of serious prospective defects early in pregnancy, and this issue of how many days will not arise.

Second, the argument from the quality of the prospective life of the defective newborn requires that we decide which defects are so serious that the kind of life the defective child can have gives it no serious claim as compared with the social costs. This issue must be thought through, and some guidelines established, but I shall not attempt this here.

One might argue that, if the newborn cannot rationally care whether its life ends or not, the parents are free to dispose of a child irrespective of whether he is defective, if they simply do not want it. To this there are two replies. First, in practice there are others who want a child if the parents do not, and they can put it up for adoption. But second, the parents are *injuring* a child if they prevent it from having the good life it could have had. We do not in general accept the argument that a person is free to injure another, for no reason, even if he has that person's consent. In view of these facts, we may expect that rational, benevolent persons deciding which moral code to support would select one that required respect for the life of a normal child, but would permit the termination of the life of a seriously defective child.

ACTIVE AND PASSIVE PROCEDURES

There is a final question: that of a choice between withdrawal of life-supporting measures (such as feeding), and the active, painless taking of life. It seems obvious, however, that once the basic decision is made that an infant is not to receive the treatment necessary to sustain life beyond a few days, it is mere stupid cruelty to allow it to waste away gradually in a hospital bed—for the child to suffer, and for everyone involved also to suffer in watching the child suffer. If death is the outcome decided upon, it is far kinder for it to come quickly and painlessly.

Notes

1. Here I disagree with Michael Tooley, "Abortion and Infanticide," *Philosophy and Public Affairs* 2 (1972): 37-65, especially pp. 44-49.

2. Professor P. Foot has made interesting remarks on when a life is worth living. See her "Euthanasia," *Philosophy and Public Affairs* 6 (1977): 85-112, especially pp. 95-96. She suggests that a good life must "contain a minimum of basic goods," although not necessarily a favorable balance of good over evil elements. When does she think this minimum fails? For one thing, in extreme senility or severe brain damage. She also cites as examples of conditions for minimal goods that "a man is not driven to work far beyond his capacity; that he has the support of a family or community; that he can more or less satisfy his hunger; that he has hopes for the future; that he can lie down to rest at night." Overwhelming pain or nausea, or crippling depression, she says, also can make life not worth living. All of these, of course, except for cases of senility and brain damage, are factors fixing whether stretches of living are highly unpleasant.

If a person thinks that life is not good unless it realizes certain human potentialities, he will think life can be bad even if liked—and so far sets a higher standard than the happiness criterion. But Foot and such writers may say that even when life is not pleasant on balance, it can still be good if human potentialities are being realized or these basic minimal conditions are met; and in that sense they set a lower standard.

3. Richard B. Brandt, "The Morality of Abortion," in an earlier form in *The Monist* 56 (1972): 504-526, and in revised form in R. L. Perkins, ed., *Abortion: Pro and Con* (Cambridge, Mass.: Schenkman Publishing Co., 1974).

4. See A. M. Shaw and I. A. Shaw, in S. Gorovitz, et al., *Moral Problems in Medicine* (Englewood Cliffs, N.J.: Prentice-Hall, Inc., 1976), pp. 335-341.

5. See, for instance, Philippa Foot, "Euthanasia," especially pp. 109-111. She writes: "So it is not for their sake but to avoid trouble to others that they are allowed to die. When brought out into the open this seems unacceptable; at least we do not easily accept the principle that adults who need special care should be counted too burdensome to be kept alive." I would think that "to avoid trouble to others" is hardly the terminology to describe the havoc that is apt to be produced. I agree that adults should not be allowed to die, or actively killed, without their consent, possibly except when they cannot give consent but are in great pain; but the reasons that justify different behavior in the two situations have appeared in the section, "Consent."

II.
RELATED ISSUES

Laila Williamson

Infanticide: An Anthropological Analysis.[1]

Infanticide is a practice present-day westerners regard as a cruel and inhuman custom, resorted to by only a few desperate and primitive people living in harsh environments. We tend to think of it as an exceptional practice, to be found only among such peoples as the Eskimos and Australian Aborigines, who are far removed in both culture and geographical distance from us and our civilized ancestors. The truth is quite different. Infanticide has been practiced on every continent and by people on every level of cultural complexity, from hunters and gatherers to high civilizations, including our own ancestors. Rather than being an exception, then, it has been the rule.[2]

A custom which is so widely distributed, both geographically and historically, must have practical functions that explain its persistence through time. This paper is an examination of the characteristics and functions of infanticide in cultures throughout the world, primarily as reported in anthropological literature. Although the treatment of infanticide in literature is uneven and varies considerably in detail, there is enough information to establish that infanticide has in its way satisfied important familial, economic, and societal needs. The control of population as an adjustment to the environmental and economic resources of both the family and the society appears to be the most prominent function. Other reasons for the practice of infanticide will also be discussed, as well as its practical value as a method to limit family size.[3]

LAILA WILLIAMSON

The practice of infanticide is often difficult to detect. Although it was carried on openly on a large scale in the Mediterranean area in antiquity and in Imperial China, as well as among the Australian Aborigines, Tikopia of Oceania, and Eskimos,[4] in most societies it is done quietly by the mother or other close relative with no further discussion on the matter. If the death is reported at all, it is listed in the category of stillbirth or accident. In this form it is unlikely to be recognized as infanticide. As a result, Human Relations Area Files include several cases for which one observer reports that infanticide is practiced, while another, speaking of the same people, states that it never occurs. Moreover, negative reports may simply reflect the fact that informants, knowing the Europeans' distaste for infanticide, preferred to echo that view, denying the practice.

Much of the ethnographic literature fails to mention either the presence or absence of infanticide. When ethnographers note this custom at all it is generally only to cite its presence. Two investigators succeeded in finding information on infanticide in ethnographers' reports for 393 societies.[5] Of these, 302 practiced infanticide at least occasionally and 91 reportedly did not. However, the authors point out that this positive evidence, particularly of preferential female infanticide, found in the ethnographic literature is only "the tip of the iceberg."[6] Many societies that deny practicing infanticide show remarkably skewed pre-adolescent sex ratios, usually in favor of males. The normal sex ratio at birth, about 105 males to 100 females, generally evens out in early childhood through the slightly higher death rate of boys. Pre-adolescent sex ratios clearly favoring males are an indirect indication of preferential female infanticide, perhaps in a covert form, as through neglect.[7] It may be that observers frequently report cases of neglect but, failing to recognize them as infanticide, they state that no infanticide is practiced in the society.

It is sometimes difficult to decide what acts constitute infanticide. Defining it as the deliberate killing of a child in its infancy, up to two years of age, covers the majority of cases. However, the line between abortion and infanticide is not always clear. The Kamchadal of northeastern Siberia, for example, have practitioners who specialize in killing a fetus through the wall of the abdomen, during the last stages of pregnancy.[8] This may result in a stillbirth or in the birth of an injured but living infant that is killed forthwith. The Yanomamö Indians of Venezuela do the same at an earlier stage in a pregnancy, during the sixth or seventh month. Is this abortion or infanticide?[9] Another blurred line exists between deliberate killing and neglect that causes the death of an infant.

Death through neglect is here classified as infanticide, despite the fact that the participants often deny, sometimes quite truthfully, any intention of killing.

Primitive abortion techniques are either relatively ineffective or dangerous. Hence, without effective contraceptive devices, sexual abstinence and infanticide were the only sure methods of controlling family size. Abstinence in the form of celibacy has been practiced occasionally with demographic effects, as, for instance, in eighteenth and nineteenth century Europe.[10] Prolonged postpartum sexual abstinence together with a long period of lactation also lowers fertility;[11] but, although it is a custom in many primitive societies, people seldom follow this rule for as long as two or three years.

A cross-cultural survey of abortion concluded that this practice was virtually universal.[12] Sometimes it is successful, and if not, the attempts usually end in infanticide as the last resort. Abortion techniques, such as the use of magic, may be harmless though ineffective; or they may be crude, mechanical methods, such as stomping on the abdomen or inserting foreign objects into the uterus. The latter may injure the woman seriously, even fatally. Infanticide is a safer method for the woman, who is a more valuable member of society than a newborn infant, and it has the added advantage of allowing the family or the society to select infants of one sex rather than the other.[13] Societies, such as the Eskimos, Yanomamö, Fiji Islanders, and Imperial China, that strongly favor children of one sex, almost always male, prefer infanticide to abortion, as do some tribes of western India, the high castes of which allow extremely few female infants to survive.[14]

In most societies children are greatly desired, and childless marriages and barren women are often objects of pity or scorn. Yet abortion and infanticide are virtually universal. A society with a strong pro-fertility ideology may at the same time condone or even sanction infanticide. Unrestrained fertility is clearly not perceived as beneficial by either societies or individuals.

We tend to think that primitive peoples who practice infanticide show a lack of love, even cruelty, towards children. However, killing a newborn is often explained as a caring act, done to save the life of an older sibling who is too young to be weaned but is already a member of the social group and cherished as such. Most primitive people love and want children, and they are more patient and indulgent with them than are parents in western societies. They disapprove of spanking and other "ill" treatment which we accept as commonplace with our children. The individuals who carry out the act of infanticide, generally parturient women, often do not like doing it, but feel they have no choice. The killing is made easier by cultural belief that a child is not fully human until accepted as a member of the social group. This acceptance may take place when the child is named, or when it appears strong enough to survive, or when it shows "human" characteristics, such as walking and talking. The time varies from a few days to several years after birth. The Peruvian Amahuaca, for instance, do not consider children fully human until they are about three years old.[15] The psychological burden of infanticide may be eased also by belief in the eventual rebirth of a killed infant. The aborigines of Groote Eylandt, Australia, for example, believe that the spirit of a dead infant goes to a store of spirit children to await rebirth, and thus the infant continues to live, although in a different form.[16]

Societies that have commonly practiced infanticide are not necessarily more cruel or violent than others. They may be violent, as are the Yanomamö, Arabs, and many others; or they may be peaceful, nonwarlike peoples like the Eskimos, Bushmen, and Tikopia. The converse is also true: several warlike African pastoral societies practice only occasional infanticide. Moreover, infanticide is seldom an expression of cruel or violent feeling. Rather, the practice is carried on for economic and demographic reasons. It is, as the Japanese term for it indicates, "weeding," like "thinning rice seedlings."[17]

Infanticide is generally carried out immediately after birth. The most common method appears to be suffocation; for example, by immediate burial, pushing the face to the ground, or drowning. Abandonment and exposure are also widely used methods. However, abandonment does not always end in death. In some societies, for instance, the Netsilik Eskimos, the infant's crying is a message to other, perhaps childless members of the group, that they may retrieve and adopt the infant if they wish. Employing a weapon or a toxic substance, such as opium, are less common methods.

No single factor can explain infanticide in all societies. It serves many different functions, several of which may operate in one society. Some of these functions are: eliminating defectives, motherless infants, multiple births, and illegitimates; spacing children; regulating future adult sex ratios; and population control.[18]

Infanticide may be widespread in a society or happen only occasionally, but it has very few, if any, exceptions with one class of infants, that is, deformed infants. The reasons for eugenic infanticide seem obvious: unwillingness or inability to assume the burden of caring for such an infant, whose future at best would be unsure.[19] The same is true of infants who are clearly "different," as, for instance, those with unusual skin color, too light or too dark.

If a mother dies in childbirth or shortly thereafter, her infant is frequently buried. Earlier, very small children had almost no chance of survival without mother's milk and care. Wet-nurses were customary in a few societies but they were not available for everybody.

Although the treatment of twins ranges from infanticide to seeing them as an exceptionally good omen, eliminating multiple births, including one or both twins, is quite common in many societies, from hunting and gathering peoples to high civilizations. The origin of removing multiple births may well be found in the inability of a woman in a nomadic society to care for more than one infant at a time.[20] If one twin is kept, it is usually a boy, or the first born if both are of the same sex. A society's ideology often re-enforces the custom of twin infanticide with a belief that twins are conceived through intercourse with an evil spirit (the Piaroa of Venezuela),[21] or that they are evidence of the mother's infidelity (the Indians of Guianas).[22] The mother may also be likened to litter-bearing animals and encounter ridicule (the Trobriand Islanders, Oceania), or repugnance (the Ibo, West Africa).[23]

The common aversion all over the world to the birth of twins has some exceptions. The Mohave Indians and other Yuman tribes of the southwestern United States, the West African Ashanti, and the East African Shilluk all consider the birth of twins a good omen and the twins themselves supernatural beings. The Balinese of Indonesia think twins of mixed sex are of divine origin, but only if born to high caste parents. The Papago of southwestern United States believe twins have magical powers like shamans.

Although there are some societies in which illegitimacy poses no serious problem, the birth of a child who has no socially accepted father, as defined in each culture, is disapproved of in most societies. If the mother has no husband, or the husband has rejected her or her child, or if the father is known or suspected to be someone other than the husband, the mother often resorts to abortion or infanticide. An illegitimate child does not have a proper place in many societies. In a patrilineal system especially, a child without a father has no lineage or clan affiliation, and is therefore often treated as an outcast.

One class of illegitimates that are almost always rejected are half-breeds. In addition to their illegitimacy, some peoples object to the "racial impurity" which they see as unattractive. Another, and by no means unimportant, reason is that many halfbreeds are the accidental result of prostitution.[24]

During the preagricultural Paleolithic period, which comprises almost 99 percent of human history, infanticide was probably universal. On the basis of archeological evidence from Paleolithic burial sites and analogy drawn from modern hunter-gatherers, the infanticide rate in the Pleistocene has been estimated as from 15 to 50 percent of live births.[25] An estimated infanticide rate of from 15 to 20 percent is given for the modern hunter-horticultural Yanomamö.[26]

Population growth was slow during the Pleistocene. Since hunter-gatherers generally enjoy good health and have relatively low natural infant mortality rates,[27] high natural infant mortality cannot account for the near stability of the population during this long period. On the other hand, high death rates for children are found among sedentary, agricultural peoples who live under conditions that favor the spread of epidemic diseases and who suffer from malnutrition due to their often protein-poor, grain-based diets. By contrast, epidemic diseases do not spread easily among dispersed hunter-gatherers, and their diets of meat and wild vegetables provide them with better nutrition.

It has been suggested that the main mechanism in stabilizing human population during the Pleistocene was infanticide,[28] probably preferential female infanticide.[29] The motivation for this practice was most likely the spacing of children, rather than any conscious effort toward population control. As a result, however, it did help in maintaining populations in harmony with their food and water resources. Decisions of whether or not to keep an infant were probably made by the mother, perhaps in consultation with her husband, and must have been based on the circumstances of the nuclear family, the number, sex, and age of older siblings. The demands of mobility do not allow a woman to breastfeed, care for, and carry more than one child at a time since she also transports the family baggage.[30] An older sibling must be weaned before a newborn can be cared for, as premature weaning endangers a child's life. A mother in this situation feels that her responsibility is to save the older sibling, and until it is strong enough to be weaned, disposing of the newborn is a necessary and benign act.

Hunter-gatherers space their children from three to five years apart. This is accomplished partly by a short period of postpartum sexual abstinence (one year or less) and by the effects of full breastfeeding. Lactation offers considerable protection against conception for about a year.[31] Any child born too soon, before the older sibling is ready for weaning, is killed.[32]

Some nomadic hunters who practice infanticide in order to space children or to limit family size, also select for the sex of infants. Among most hunter-gatherers, women, who do most of the gathering, actually provide the bulk of the group's food from steady and reliable vegetable resources. Yet, as the prevalence of female infanticide shows, when one sex is favored over the other it is almost always the male. Very few cases of preferential male infanticide are known.[33] A people disposing of female infants may give ideological explanations for the practice, often expressing high regard for males and low regard for females. But whatever the reasons given, the effect of female infanticide is to check population growth, since removing female infants, potential child bearers, is more effective than male deaths in limiting births.[34]

Female infanticide is common in societies where a high death rate among men would otherwise create an imbalance in adult sex ratios. The high adult male death rate may be a result of extensive warfare, as among the hunter-horticultural Yanomamö, or be due to other dangers to men, such as hunting accidents among the Eskimos.

The Eskimos strongly prefer male children who are the future hunters. Since there are no vegetable foods to collect in the long arctic winters, the hunters are virtually the sole providers of food. It is therefore particularly important for Eskimo parents to have boys. Breastfeeding and caring for a female infant would delay the birth and raising of a boy. It is felt that several boys should be growing up before any girls are accepted. An Eskimo hunter's life is dangerous and many die young in hunting accidents. Without female infanticide the adult sex ratio would become unbalanced, and there would be too few hunters to provide for the women and children. The result would be starvation and death for adults as well as children.

Many aboriginal peoples have successfully adjusted their population size to the available food supply. The Tikopia are an example of a horticultural group living in a state of equilibrium with their food resources in a well-functioning social system. In this instance the principal means of population control were infanticide, celibacy, and suicidal sea voyages by young men. The Tikopia live on a small Polynesian island, subsisting on vegetable crops, fish, and other marine resources.[35] The cultivated land was traditionally divided among families. In order to prevent the division of the gardens, from which the extended family derived their vegetable products, into ever smaller holdings, the eldest son inherited the land. A younger brother should not have children and was often expected to remain unmarried. Married couples had on the average 3.5 children.[36] Newborn infants in excess of the number of children deemed right by the head of the family were put to death at birth. Both sexes were killed, but perhaps slightly more males were kept.[37] The Tikopia were themselves aware of the delicate balance between population and resources, and were concerned about the consequences of interference by Europeans.[38] The upsetting of an economic and social system, which would bring suffering and misery to many, was more wrong to the Tikopia than quietly disposing of superfluous infants.[39]

Some societies with ranked castes have practiced infanticide in order to keep genealogical lines pure and for other reasons of status. The Tahitians, for example, killed the infants of couples of unequal rank.[40] Among the royal family of old Uganda all children born to daughters of a king were killed, as well as the sons of royal wives whose offspring were ineligible to succeed the king. An extreme case of status infanticide was found among the high caste Jhareja Rajputs of northwestern India who killed almost all female infants at birth.[41] The families in this highest caste thus avoided paying large dowries and wedding expenses. Instead, by having only sons who married women of lower castes, they were the recipients of dowries. In this system the wealth kept moving up to the highest caste.

Infanticide has been customary in high civilizations as well as primitive and small scale societies. In Imperial China, Japan, and Europe it was used as a method of controlling population growth and avoiding starvation and social disruption. It was very widespread in China up to the time of the Communist Revolution. When limits of the arable land and food production capacity were reached, the population had to be stabilized. Infanticide was the main mechanism of population control, although late age of marriage and abortion were also customary to a lesser degree. Females were not valued and were selected for infanticide first, as males were preferred to perpetuate the family line. The decision for or against keeping an infant was made by the male head of the family at the birth of the child or even before. A family might raise two sons but, at most, one daughter, who would be later exchanged for a wife for one of the sons. During famines caused by drought, floods, earthquakes, and such, female infanticide reached even higher proportions, resulting in a shortage of women later on. Sometimes as many as a quarter of the marriageable men in the peasant class could not find a wife. This was a direct result of female infanticide and was instrumental in reducing the population even further. Also, in times of famine or exceptionally high taxes small girls were subjected to mortal neglect, and older ones were sold into slavery or prostitution to relieve the burden on the family's reduced resources.

In classical Greece and Rome infanticide was accepted as a matter of course, and very few contemporary voices were raised against it.[42] Families might keep two or three sons, as males were preferred, but rarely more than one daughter.[43] In fact, infanticide was considered such a natural and commonplace event that it was an accepted topic for humor in the comedies of the time.[44]

The main reasons for infanticide in antiquity as well as in medieval and later times appear to have been poverty and periodic famines. There were no meaningful attempts to stop the large scale killing of infants in Europe until the latter half of the nineteenth century. In the laws of many European countries infanticide was a crime but very few people were brought to trial for it.[45] Societies accepted the custom because most people simply could not feed and care for a large number of children. By the eighteenth century there was the additional problem of the numerous illegitimate infants born to female servants and factory workers who had been sexually exploited by their employers.[46] Since such exploitation was an accepted practice, infanticide was most often the only practical alternative for these women. In the contemporary view of society infanticide was apparently preferable to holding the higher class male partners responsible.

The incidence of infanticide in Africa appears to be lower than among peoples of other continents. Africans do also eliminate defectives, usually twins, and sometimes illegitimates, although in the latter case abortion is often preferred. African hunter-gatherers (e.g., the Bushmen), some pastoralists (e.g., the Chagga of East Africa and the Malagasy of Madagascar island, who are also rice cultivators), and a few agriculturalists (e.g., the South African Bemba) practice infanticide to control population or space children. But many of the agricultural and pastoral peoples of Africa do not. Some possible reasons for this should be discussed.

Bantu-speaking agriculturalists are relatively recent arrivals in most parts of Africa. Armed with superior technology, iron tools, and a knowledge of agriculture, they rapidly spread southwards from their original home, probably in West Africa, beginning some 2000 or 1500 years ago. They were still spreading during the 1600s.[47] The earlier inhabitants, hunters and gatherers with sparse population densities, were pushed into marginal areas. Until recent decades there was plenty of arable land available to support growing populations of agriculturalists. The ready availability of land, however, is not a sufficient reason by itself to forgo or abandon the practice of infanticide. Hunter-horticulturalists of the Amazon region, for example, have traditionally had areas to move into, but they practice infanticide for other cultural reasons, such as to select for the sex of infants and to space children.

Some pastoralists, too, migrated south relatively recently from their ancestral home in northeastern Africa. They spread into only partially occupied areas, which they could exploit more intensively as pastoralists. Many of them settled into a seminomadic pattern of life, with permanent villages surrounded by gardens and with seasonal cattle camps.

A large family becomes an economic asset under agricultural and pastoral conditions by providing a large number of people to work in the fields and with the herds. The work includes tasks that even small children can perform. Frequently children of five or six start work in the fields or as herdboys. Thus the labor of small children is valued, and it is one reason why a large number of offspring are desirable. Under such circumstances infanticide would not benefit the family. On the contrary, it would deprive the parents of potential contributors to the family's wellbeing. Also, a family of many workers could more easily increase production, as was often necessary to pay taxes in colonial times.

Other factors must be considered when discussing the population dynamics of Africa. One must note, for instance, the losses in populations caused by the slave trade and the mortality that ordinarily accompanies colonial conditions. Although Africans had some immunity to Old World diseases, many still died in epidemics.

Furthermore, infant mortality in Africa is very high. It is frequently described as "extremely high"[48] or "appalling."[49] Some estimates of child mortality among several African agriculturalists and pastoralists vary from 26 percent to over 50 percent of live births.[50] A high birth rate in a population goes hand in hand with high infant mortality.[51] Most

African agricultural peoples have diets that consist primarily of grain and root crops without adequate amounts of animal protein. Under these conditions malnutrition, weanling diarrhea, and epidemic diseases take a high toll of infants and small children. A large number of children thus helps to ensure that at least a few will reach adulthood.

Yet these Africans, too, have tried to space births, primarily by postpartum sexual abstinence. This practice is considerably more widespread in Africa than in other parts of the world.[52] The custom of long postpartum sexual abstinence, lasting more than a year, is effective in reducing the number of births in a population.[53] It should also give children a better chance of survival because it allows for a longer nursing period. But the length of time between births among the sedentary Africans is apparently not long enough to ensure the survival of the older sibling in the absence of a nutritionally adequate diet. Hunter-gatherers with children spaced from three to five years apart and with better diets have infant mortality rates that are considerably lower than those of the agriculturalists and pastoralists, whose children are usually weaned around the age of two at the arrival of a new baby.

An infant or small child is in great danger at the time of weaning and many of them die of weanling diarrhea and epidemic diseases. And some of those who do survive suffer physiological damage because of malnutrition. They may only live a short life of suffering. Many agricultural and pastoral Africans have in effect opted for the more wasteful, "natural" death.

Wartime killing of infants by an enemy has been excluded from this discussion because it is part of the whole pattern of treatment of people by hostile outsiders. But there are also reports of people killing their own infants in wartime because their crying could disclose the hiding place of a group (the Tlingit of the Northwest Coast of North America, for example), or to keep them from being captured, or because of starvation (for instance, the Maori of New Zealand). Several Central American Indian groups such as the Chontal and the Indians of Haiti, all of Greater Antilles, in fact, resorted to abortions, infanticide, and even suicides to escape Spanish oppression. Harassment by Europeans is given as a reason for infanticide among the Tasmanians. Infants and small children slowed the travel speed of the adults who had to flee to avoid being murdered by Europeans.

The ritual sacrifice of infants is unlikely to have had appreciable demographic or economic effects on population because it was not practiced on a very large scale. It was common among pre-Christian Europeans and Mediterranean peoples before Greek and Roman times, as far back as the time of ancient Hebrews, Egyptians, and Babylonians.[54] Infants and children were sacrificed to propitiate gods; they were sealed in walls and buried in foundations for buildings and bridges. This kind of ritual sacrifice of infants was found among some non-European peoples too, such as the coastal Indians of southeastern North America,[55] the Chibcha of South America,[56] and the Maya and Aztec of Mexico. It occurred primarily in chiefdoms and states, seldom in small scale societies, and rarely on such a scale as among pre-Christian Mediterranean peoples, or the Aztec. Whether infant sacrifice had any significant effect on the populations of the societies practicing it is difficult to determine accurately without knowing their demographic structure. However, an estimate of the number of sacrificed infants and small children in precolonial Mexico, for example, about two thousand annually, is not considered a meaningful increase in mortality in the total population of contemporary Mexico.[57] It is unlikely that ritual infant sacrifices affected infant mortality to a significant extent for another reason; many of those who were sacrificed might well have been killed in infancy anyway.[58]

Infanticide is now considered a crime by national governments all over the world. It is true that even in our own society, despite enforced legal sanctions, the practice still occurs even if on a much reduced scale. Nevertheless, it has been abandoned as an accepted method of population control and has become the exception in western civilized societies, especially now that family size can be regulated through contraception and medically safe abortion. Moreover, the killing of infants has been abandoned by most nonwestern societies as well, for various reasons stemming from contact with representatives of western civilization.

Primitive societies everywhere have been disrupted and otherwise influenced by contact with Europeans. Very few peoples remain in aboriginal conditions today.[59] In most nonwestern societies early contacts caused severe depopulation through both exploitation and the introduction of new, epidemic diseases. In addition, the spread of venereal diseases has lowered fertility among many aboriginal peoples. After the worst initial depopulation, missionaries and colonial govenments encouraged population growth by attempting to eradicate both infanticide and abortion. Despite these and other continuing attempts to the contrary, infanticide may persist if the local community does not disapprove of it.[60] The influence of western civilization continues to increase, however, leading to an ever closer integration of primitive societies with national governments and the eventual abandoning of infanticide.

People have to contend with population problems and, as this short presentation shows, the widespread practice of infanticide throughout most of human history, and in so many different cultures, attests to its past acceptance as an effective method of population control. The reasons for infanticide have been overwhelmingly economic and demographic. The great majority of infanticides have been performed to keep the size of families and, indirectly, societies adjusted to their environmental and economic conditions. The adjustment to food resources, to the subsistence pattern of each society, or to nomadic conditions appear to be very basic reasons for infanticide, as it was the only practical and reliable method for limiting the number of children.

Notes

1. I am grateful to Dr. Gertrude E. Dole, Dr. Stanley A. Freed, Dr. Robert L. Carneiro, and Priscilla Ward for their support and helpful comments while I was writing this paper.
2. Incidence of infanticide has been reported for nonhuman primates as well. See Sarah Blaffer Hrdy, "Infanticide as a Primate Reproductive Strategy," *American Scientists* 65, no. 1 (1977): 40-49.
3. The present tense, "ethnographic present," is used in this discussion, although most societies have abandoned the practice of infanticide in recent times.
4. Unless otherwise specified, the source for information on individual societies presented in this paper is Human Relations Area Files, Institute of Human Relations, Yale University.
5. William Tulio Divale and Marvin Harris, "Population, Warfare, and the Male Supremacist Complex," *American Anthropologist* 78 (1976): 521-538, 525.
6. Ibid.
7. Ibid., pp. 525-526.
8. G. W. Steller, *Beschriebung von dem Lande Kamtschatka*, (1774), as quoted in George Devereux, *A Study of Abortion in Primitive Societies* (New York: The Julian Press, 1955), p. 252.
9. See also Mildred Dickeman, "Demographic Consequences of Infanticide in Man," *Annual Review of Ecology and Systematics* 6 (1975): 107-137, 109-110.
10. William L. Langer, "Checks on Population Growth: 1750-1850," *Scientific American* 226, no. 2 (1972): 92-99, 95.
11. Moni Nag, "Factors Affecting Human Fertility in Non-Industrial Societies: A Cross-Cultural Study," Yale University Publications in Anthropology, no. 66 (New Haven, Conn.: Yale University Publications in Anthropology, 1962), p. 79.
12. Devereux, *Study of Abortion*, p. 161.
13. Divale and Harris, "Population, Warfare, and the Male Supremacist Complex," pp. 530-531.
14. Kanti Pakrasi, *Female Infanticide in India* (Calcutta, India: Edition Indian, 1970), p. 33.
15. Dole and Carneiro, personal communication.
16. Frederick G. G. Rose, "Australian Marriage, Land-owning Groups, and Initiations," in *Man the Hunter*, ed. Richard B. Lee and Irven DeVore (Chicago, Ill.: Aldine & Atherton, 1968), pp. 200-208, p. 204.

17. Dickeman, "Demographic Consequences of Infanticide," p. 126.
18. See also Dickeman, "Demographic Consequences of Infanticide," p. 116.
19. Allan R. Holmberg, *Nomads of the Long Bow* (New York: Natural History Press, 1969), p. 174, reports that the Bolivian Sirionò do not practice any infanticide. During his fieldwork among them in 1941-42, he saw several clubfooted individuals. Unfortunately we know next to nothing of the aboriginal Sirionò culture. Holmberg was the first anthropologist to seriously study them. These people had for several decades before the 1940s been under intense influence of the missionaries and Bolivian government agencies. Several Sirionò groups, including the one Holmberg studied, lived for some time at a mission or the government Indian school and took up intermittently their traditional nomadic life (p. XXII). The fact that no infanticide was observed in the 1930s and 1940s does not preclude the possibility that it was a custom in the aboriginal Sirionò culture.
20. See also Gary Granzberg, "Twin Infanticide—A Cross-Cultural Test of a Materialistic Explanation," *Ethos* 1, no. 4 (1973): 405-412, 410-411.
21. Carneiro, personal communication.
22. Walter E. Roth, "An Introductory Study of the Arts, Crafts, and Customs of the Guiana Indians," in the *38th Annual Report of the Bureau of American Ethnology* (1916-1917), pp. 25-745, p. 558.
23. G. T. Basden, *Among the Ibos of Nigeria* (London: Seeley & Service, 1921), p. 57.
24. George Devereux, "Mohave Indian Infanticide," *The Psychoanalytic Review* 35, no. 2 (April 1948): 126-139, 128-129.
25. Joseph B. Birdsell, "Some Predictions for the Pleistocene Based on Equilibrium Systems among Hunter-Gatherers," in Lee and Devore, *Man the Hunter*, pp. 229-240, p. 239.
26. James V. Neel, "Lessons from a 'Primitive' People," *Science* 170, no. 3960 (1970): 815-822, 816.
27. Ibid.
28. Lee and Devore, *Man the Hunter*, p. 11.
29. Birdsell, "Predictions for the Pleistocene," p. 239.
30. Ibid., p. 236.
31. Jeroen K. Van Ginneken, "Prolonged Breastfeeding as a Birth Spacing Method," *Studies in Family Planning* 5 (1974): 201-208, 201; and J. Knodel and E. van de Welle, "Breastfeeding, Fertility and Infant Mortality," *Population Studies* 21, no. 2 (1967): 109-131, 114.
32. Analogies from today's marginal, remnant groups of hunter-gatherers to preagricultural human past must be made with great care. Dickeman makes this point when she discusses infanticide among the nomadic Bushmen of South Africa ("Demographic Consequences," pp. 121-122). Richard E. Lee and Nancy Howell have both recently reported that the !Kung Bushmen practice infanticide only occasionally and mainly on defectives. These reports are at variance with earlier information on the Bushmen in general by I. Schapera and by Lorna Marshall. Dickeman suggests that today's Bushmen have been increasingly affected by contact with the surrounding populations and suffered a loss of fertility through introduced diseases, especially venereal disease. The latter lowers fertility levels considerably (Nag, "Factors Affecting Fertility," pp. 123-124). These might be the reasons for a low rate of infanticide among today's Bushmen, but this low rate should not be seen as evidence for the same among Pleistocene hunters.
33. The Rendille, a group of camel herders in Kenya are one. According to Mary Douglas in "Population Control in Primitive Groups," *British Journal of Sociology* 27 (1966): 263-273, 269-270, the Rendille kill all boys born on Wednesdays and those born after the eldest brother has been circumcised. They must keep the size of their camel herds delicately adjusted to the environment, and therefore, cannot have too many sons as heirs to the herds. The male population is kept down by emigration and male infanticide.
34. This applies to all societies that practice female infanticide, not only hunters and gatherers.
35. Raymond Firth, *We, the Tikopia* (London: Allen & Unwin, 1957).
36. Ibid., p. 411.

37. Ibid., pp. 410-411.
38. Ibid., p. 417.
39. Ibid., p. 530.
40. Irving Goldman, *Ancient Polynesian Society* (Chicago, Ill.: Chicago University Press, 1970), p. 563.
41. Pakrasi, *Female Infanticide*, p. 33.
42. William L. Langer, "Infanticide: A Historical Survey," *History of Childhood Quarterly* 1, no. 3 (1974): 353-365, 354-355; and Lloyd DeMause, *The Evolution of Childhood* (New York: The Psychohistory Press, 1974), p. 26.
43. Langer, "Infanticide," p. 354; DeMause, *Evolution of Childhood*, p. 26.
44. For instance, Menander, "The Girl from Samos" and "The Arbitration," trans. L. A. Post in *The Complete Greek Drama*, vol. II, ed. Whitney J. Oates and Eugene O'Neill, Jr. (New York: Random House, 1938).
45. Langer, "Infanticide," pp. 355-356.
46. Ibid., p. 357.
47. Simon and Phoebe Ottenberg, *Cultures and Societies of Africa* (New York: Random House, 1960), p. 71.
48. Ibid., p. 17. Remy Clairin calls both infant and child (up to age five) mortality rates in Africa extremely high ("The Assessment of Infant and Child Mortality from the Data Available in Africa," in *The Population of Tropical Africa*, ed. J. C. Caldwell, and C. Okonjo [London: Longman, 1968], p. 199).
49. J. A. Massam, *The Cliff Dwellers of Kenya* (London: Seeley & Service, 1921), p. 168.
50. D. I. Roberts, "A Demographic Study of a Dinka Village," *Human Biology* 28, no. 3 (1956): 323-349, 339.
51. Neel, "Lessons from a Primitive People," p. 817.
52. Jean-Francois Saucier, "Correlates of the Long Postpartum Taboo: A Cross-Cultural Study," *Current Anthropology* 13, no. 2 (1972): 238-249, 243. Steven Polgar, in the same issue of *Current Anthropology*, p. 206, suggests on the basis of Saucier's work that the custom of long postpartum sexual abstinence may postdate the agricultural revolution. In that case the preagricultural ancestors of African cultivators may have practiced infanticide more commonly, too. However, we have no evidence either way.
53. Nag, "Factors Affecting Fertility," p. 79.
54. DeMause, *Evolution of Childhood*, p. 27; and James Hastings, ed., *Encyclopedia of Religion and Ethics* (New York: Charles Scribner's Sons, n.d.), vol. 6, p. 32, pp. 840-867.
55. Harold E. Driver, *Indians of North America* 2nd ed. (Chicago: Chicago University Press, 1969), p. 325.
56. Alfred E. Kroeber, "The Chibcha," in *Handbook of South American Indians*, ed. Julian Steward, Bulletin of the Bureau of American Ethnology 143 (Washington D.C.: Government Printing Office, 1946), vol. 2, pp. 887-909, p. 907.
57. S. F. Cook, "Human Sacrifice and Warfare as Factors in the Demography of Pre-Colonial Mexico," *Human Biology* 18, no. 2 (1946): 81-99, 85-86.
58. Infants were purchased from their mothers for sacrifice, for example, in pre-colonial Mexico (Cook, "Human Sacrifice and Warfare," p. 85), India (*Encyclopedia of Religion and Ethics*, vol. 6, p. 850), and in Carthage (Plutarch *Moralia*, as quoted in DeMause, *Evolution of Childhood*, p. 27).
59. The Yanomamö who practice infanticide are among the few societies which have experienced relatively little interference from missionaries or national governments thus far.
60. For example, Yolanda and Robert Murphy have reported on the continuing occurrence of infanticide among the Mundurucù Indians of Brazil, despite strenuous efforts of missionaries to eradicate the practice (Yolanda and Robert Murphy, *Women of the Forest* [New York: Columbia University Press, 1974], pp. 165-166).

Brandt F. Steele

Psychology of Infanticide Resulting from Maltreatment

There are many ways in which infants are killed, and complex variations in the psychology of the caretakers who are instrumental in causing their death. Death of an infant or child as the result of maltreatment is one extreme of the broad spectrum of child abuse and neglect. It merges almost imperceptibly into other forms of infanticide that are related to economic, moral, religious, political, or military causes or to culturally determined superstitions and personal vendettas. A common denominator of all such variations, including maltreatment, is the assumption that the rights, desires, and ideas of the adult take full precedence over those of the child, and that children are essentially the property of parents who have the right to deal with their offspring as they see fit, without interference. Such concepts are deeply imbedded in human history and have persisted through the centuries despite recurrent and increasing attempts to establish the rights of the child.

It is useful to differentiate the direct murder of children without pre-existing maltreatment from the killing of infants as a result of recurrent abuse. In the former, death is brought about by an acutely or chronically psychotic parent, relative, or acquaintance. The child has been taken into

This article is derived from work done over several years, and partially supported at different times by The Childrens Bureau, The Commonwealth Fund, The Grant Foundation, The Kaiser Family Foundation, and The Robert Wood Johnson Foundation.

76

the system of delusions and hallucinations of the psychotic adult and is then perceived as a dangerous or evil object that must be eradicated. The child is attacked with the clear purpose of murder. Occasionally the "voice of God" is heard directing the death of the child, and there is a pseudoaltruistic type, in which a severely depressed parent will kill self and children to "prevent suffering and unhappiness."

Caretakers, most often parents, whose repeated abuse of a child results in death do not, as a rule, have any intent to kill. On the contrary, they have an investment in a living child who should be well behaved and satisfy parental demands. The abuse is essentially excessive physical punishment designed to make the child stop bad behavior and alter his ways so as to please the parent. The fact that death occurs is rather "accidental," unintentional, and often the cause of some dismay. The parent may feel great guilt and sadness and deeply mourn the loss of the child, or may sometimes defensively rationalize the death as another evidence of the child's defectiveness, contrariness, or even malicious intent to create trouble. Not rarely, parents deny any actions which could have contributed to their child's death, blaming it on unknown accidental causes, or even blaming all the injuries found at autopsy on the resuscitation efforts made by doctors and nurses in the emergency room.

Parents and other caretakers who have the pattern of abusing or neglecting their infants come from all walks of life and have about the same kinds and degrees of neuroses and emotional problems as the rest of the general population. Independent of the presence or absence of any significant mental health problems they share a number of psychological traits, beliefs, and attitudes; and they almost invariably have a history of significant emotional and physical neglect with varying amounts of physical abuse in their earliest years. As noted above, they have a firm conviction that parental rights and needs far outweigh those of infants. In addition, they have a strong belief in the educational value and necessity of physical punishment, and in stern discipline in general, with a corresponding fear of the baby getting "spoiled" even in the first few months of life. They seem to misperceive the infant as older, wiser, and more capable than he really is, expecting efficient response and action much too soon in the infant's life. Inevitably the infant fails; the corrective punishment is applied. There is also a significant lack of empathic awareness of the infant's fluctuating state and needs and a corresponding lack of sensitive, appropriate caretaking responses to them. The parent responds in ways that suit his or her own whims and convenience rather than to the child's specific wants. As a general rule, the more aggression and violence experienced in the earliest family setting, the greater will be the tendency to use violence in later life, even to the point of killing a child. The more kindness and understanding experienced with parents or other persons, the more these qualities will appear in later parenting behavior. The identifications with the early models of parenting behavior and with the authoritative figures of infancy have lasting effects, which surface in later life. Correspondingly, the abuser often sees his own bad childhood self reincarnated in his infant, who is therefore punished for the same unsatisfactory behavior for which the parent received punishment. Such perceptions of the child are often highly erroneous, being projections rather than accurate evaluations.

Such beliefs, attitudes, and behaviors evidenced by abusive parents are with few exceptions essentially repetitions of the way their own parents took care of them in their earliest years, although many people cannot consciously recall those events. The basic, emotionally tinged ingredients of parenting behavior seem to be learned in the first three years of life; only the mechanical aspects of parent craft are learned at later times. Just as good parents repeat the devoted empathic care of their early years, so do abusive parents repeat the unhappy patterns of their own early experiences.

There are other residues of their early years that plague abusers. Prominent is a tragically low sense of self-esteem and feeling of inability to ever do anything well enough, although this is sometimes hidden under a defensive veneer of overweening self-confidence and braggadocio. Closely allied is a difficult-to-assuage dependent need for care and understanding, accompanied by an equally potent lack of basic trust and fear of trying to seek either pleasure or help from other adults. Unfortunately, such people tend to follow a pattern of assortive mating, and marry or live with others very much like themselves, equally deprived and needy, with no store of surplus love or understanding to draw on in time of crisis. They lead lonely lives, isolated emotionally, if not geographically, from family and friends, feeling they must solve all their problems without outside aid. It is not surprising under these circumstances that the abuser, in times of stress, has no place to turn for reassurance or comfort except to the infant. If the infant's response or behavior is not sufficiently rewarding or "approving" of parental actions, the caretaker can release punitive anger with a sense of righteous indignation at the spoiled, ungrateful, naughty child. Such situations also provide the channel for the discharge of anger originally felt toward frustrating, unresponsive, unloving parents. Punishment easily escalates into abuse with injury to the infant, and, if repeated enough or severe enough, can cause death.

Because of their own inadequate coping abilities plus their inability to seek help, abusers are particularly vulnerable to crises in their lives. They are easily thrown into difficulty by marital problems, mild friction in any other of their fragile interpersonal relationships, or by increase in long-standing intrapsychic states of depression and anxiety. There may be devastating problems related to poverty, unemployment, alcoholism, poor housing, or the breakdown of appliances and automobiles. Such environmental disasters, while potent exacerbators of trouble, are not essential instigators of abuse; it is well-known that abuse and infanticide also occur in significant numbers in upper socioeconomic levels, despite good housing, education, employment, and lack of alcohol. The most commonly perceived stress to which the caretaker responds is the misbehaving infant, the one who cries too much or too long, does not eat properly or messes food, soils at the wrong time or in the wrong place, is too active or too quiet, is too vocal or too dumb, or is generally disobedient. To a neutral outside observer such behaviors might well seem to be within the limits of normal infant activities, or at least something that could be managed by some means other than abuse. But to the abusive parent they are overwhelming, because the infant is failing to meet the impossibly high expectations placed upon it.

Although abusive caretakers in general share the same kind of backgrounds, psychological patterns, and child-rearing practices, there is a wide range in the severity and frequency of their violent behaviors, even among those who eventually kill a child. The following highly condensed case histories demonstrate three of the many possible variations of the main themes.

Mr. and Mrs. A. had three children, Lisa, age 4, Joe, age 2½ from her previous marriage, and Billy, age 1, from their present union. Mrs. A. had been mildly physically abused by her father and emotionally rejected by mother as well as by father and four brothers. She was a lonely, depressed, isolated person with a low sense of self-worth. She had divorced her first husband because he did not support her, drank heavily, took drugs, and was abusive to her and their two babies. Joe, named after his father, had been repeatedly abused and neglected, failed to thrive, was placed in foster care for several months and then returned to his mother. He was developmentally behind schedule due to deprivation, but not seriously retarded. He had problems around feeding and was not toilet trained.

Mr. A. had grown up in a chaotic family and neighborhood, exposed to considerable familial and environmental violence. He had some trust in a sister, but in no one else in the world, not even his mother, who he felt used him but never really cared for him. He said he saw the world differently than anyone else and dealt with it aggressively, often getting in fights, losing jobs, drinking, and having minor brushes with the law. He frequently punished all three children, causing moderate bruising, for failing to obey or behave. He was especially incensed by Joey soiling his pants and bed and eating improperly; he frequently punished him severely, as did Mrs. A. in milder form.

One day after Mr. A. came home in a bad humor following a short stay in jail for a minor offense, he became very angry over Joey's soiling and beat him more than usual. Soon afterwards Joe was dead on arrival at the hospital, and the autopsy showed multiple bruises, ruptured intestine, and brain injury.

The case of Mr. and Mrs. A. and Joe is fairly typical of the more flagrant types of repeated abuse culminating in death. Mr. A. falls into the classification of sociopathic character. His violence is widespread and he has no real regard for other human beings. Such persons, although they often come to the attention of authorities and agencies, constitute only a small percentage of child abusers. The following case is quite similar to the preceding one in the facts of what happened. But the parents are quite different from the A.'s.

Mr. and Mrs. B. had three children, Andy, age 5, Carla, age 3, and Sally, 1½. Mrs. B. was one of five siblings, all of whom were physically abused by both parents. She and her mother had been at odds all her life, and her mother often refused to see her for months at a time. Mr. B. and his brother had been severely abused by their father, with many minor injuries. Their mother was also attacked, especially if she tried to protect her boys. In addition to other kinds of abuse, the father used to kick Mr. B. in the back and stomach with his pointed cowboy boots. Mr. B.'s sister "could get away with anything" and was never punished.

Both Mr. and Mrs. B. believed in strict discipline to insure obedience and good behavior, and severe spanking of the children, including Sally, was routine.

Carla was singled out for especially severe punishment by both parents, but particularly by Mr. B., who was very concerned lest she be "spoiled." This pattern was exacerbated by Mr. B.'s father, who on frequent visits gave attention and favors to Carla and occasionally abused Andy. Once when Mr. B. spanked Carla for creating a disturbance at a family holiday dinner, his father attacked him with his fists. Over a period of many months Carla suffered severe bruises, a couple of minor fractures, lacerations, and serious burns. After a short period in protective foster care she was returned to parental custody.

One night Carla was brought to a hospital emergency room, moribund. Autopsy revealed multiple bruises, ruptured intestine, peritonitis, pneumonia, and brain injury. No immediate precipitating crisis in the family could be ascertained, but some months later Mr. B. revealed he had on several occasions kicked Carla in the stomach, much as his father had kicked him.

This case shows how childhood abuse and specific conflictual intrafamily relationships can be revived in adult years and influence abusive parental behavior, with specific bearing on the idiosyncratic meaning of a certain child, as well as a particular style of abuse. Mr. and Mrs. B. were good average citizens. They were devout churchgoers, buying their home and making wise real-estate investments. He occasionally drank, not to excess, and was a steady, skilled, highly valued blue-collar worker. Yet they were plagued by feelings of poor self-esteem and, except for some relatives, had few friends and led a rather isolated life. Rarely did they do anything for pleasure.

A third case, again similar in its outcome, demonstrates another variant of the problem.

Mr. and Mrs. C. had two children, David, 4½, and Lucy, 3½. They had come from another state and had no nearby relatives and few close friends. Mr. C. had been raised somewhat haphazardly, without a father most of the time but without any significant neglect and only an "average amount of spanking." He was a quiet, aloof, uncommunicative kind of person, not at all demonstrative or supportive with his wife. Mrs. C.'s father had left when she was 6, and she never had a stepfather. Her mother worked and she took over much of the care of her five-year-younger brother, whom she loved dearly. She was the focus of her mother's concern and demand, did a lot of the housework, made excellent grades in school, and was a regular church attendant. Her older sisters did little work, lived loosely, left school, but were not much criticized nor punished. Mrs. C. herself would never dare be disobedient or talk back, lest her mother whip her.

Both Mr. and Mrs. C. gave preference to David and only spanked him moderately. Mr. C. liked him because he was the first born, a son, and named after him. Mrs. C. saw in him the duplicate of her dearly loved little brother, whom she had raised. Both parents were generally good and quite loving toward David.

Mr. C. was almost equally loving toward Lucy, and "let her get away with things," which annoyed his wife. Mrs. C. also loved Lucy and was generally quite motherly with her. However, if Lucy seemed to be getting extra favors or was not behaving properly, Mrs. C. would seem to see her as the early life sisters who went free while she herself slaved and took the brunt of things. At such times she would spank and hit Lucy, sometimes hard enough to cause a bruise.

In late October Mrs. C. bought candy in preparation for Halloween "trick or treat." She put it away and told the children very firmly not to touch it. Later, on returning home from errands, she found her husband had given both children some of the candy and they were happily eating it. She thought Lucy was enjoying not only the candy but also evading mother's command. Mrs. C. felt quite put down and angry, hit Lucy fairly hard several times with her hand and with a stick. Lucy accidentally fell onto the sharp corner of the coffee table. Later in the evening she became quite ill, and was taken to the hospital where she soon died. Autopsy revealed a few bruises, a ruptured liver with massive hemorrhage, and fractures of four ribs.

The C.'s are a solid, lower middle-class family. Both of them work and go to school to advance their skills. They are financially stable and responsible, have two cars, and are buying a home in a nice neighborhood. Yet they do not do much as a family in the way of recreation, and Mrs. C. particularly does almost nothing for the sake of pleasure. She still works very hard, doing her proper duty as she was taught to do. She tried to make her daughter do as she was made to do, and punished her as she would have been punished as a child for doing wrong. She also released some of the anger harbored against her sisters. Lucy's death was, in a sense, purely accidental. But it did occur during the process of more than averagely intense punishment or abuse.

Maltreatment resulting in death is not always an expression of physical abuse. It can also be related to neglect, a type of distorted parenting in which the caretaker fails to provide material care in the form of food, clothing, cleanliness, and basic medical care, or enough sensory and motor stimulation for the infant. These failures may in some cases be due to poverty or inescapable environmental problems, but it is rare in our society for devoted parents to be unable to find some way, through public or private agencies, of providing minimal care for their babies. Neglect is almost always due to a clear inability of the parent, for psychological reasons, to carry out the basic minimum of caretaking tasks. This inability is manifested in the lack of empathic sensitivity to both perceive the child's state and needs and respond appropriately to them. It includes what we commonly call "maternal deprivation."

As a rule, parents who neglect their offspring are very similar to those who abuse. They have had the same experience of being poorly parented in early years and show the same psychological patterns. In fact, although abuse and neglect may each exist in pure culture, it is not rare for parents to both abuse and neglect the same child at different times, or to abuse one child and neglect another of their infants. In somewhat simplified terms the chief difference between abuse and neglect lies in the final behavior of a parent who perceives the infant as unsatisfactory or misbehaving in some way. The parent may decide the only appropriate measure is to punish the child to make it "shape up," in which case there will be abuse. On the other hand, the parent may decide it is a hopeless task, the infant is beyond help, too worthless and unrewarding to bother with; there is no longer any point in caring for it or about it, and the picture of neglect ensues. In general, neglecting caretakers, mostly mothers, tend to be more depressed, listless, hopeless, and more isolated, with their aggression more deeply submerged than is usual in abusive parents.

In a minority of cases the depression is of psychotic proportions. The mother is nearly immobilized and so deeply out of contact with reality she is hardly aware she even has a baby. After varying amounts of neglect, she may, under influence of her psychotic delusions, kill her baby. The syndrome of postpartum depression is recognized as a frequent cause of infanticide. Sometimes a parent who is mentally retarded will neglect an infant with fatal results, not out of any malicious intent, but because of cognitive inability to keep track of necessary caretaking tasks. Schizophrenia, too, can in some cases seriously interfere with caretaking; in psychotic withdrawn states the parent can completely forget the existence of the child. We knew a rather well-compensated schizophrenic young woman who moved with her husband and small baby to live in a trailer in an isolated area totally away from her supportive family and friends. She gradually decompensated and became increasingly withdrawn and less able to cope. Her husband was insensitive to this problem and did not help. One morning, standing and looking at a T.V. program in an almost trancelike state, she let the baby slip out of her arms and hit the floor on its head. The baby died of skull fracture and hemorrhage in the brain.

A very common manifestation of neglect is known as "failure to thrive due to maternal deprivation." In such cases the emaciation and arrested physical and emotional development cannot be explained by any recognized disease. Such infants begin to thrive when brought into the hospital or placed in good foster homes. Usually there is accompanying physical neglect, the child being dirty, listless, generally uncared for, and very susceptible to infections. If not recognized and treated, the infant will die of malnutrition and intercurrent infectious disease. Another type of neglect is that in which the infant is materially well cared for, fed, and clothed in a clean environment, but is deprived of adequate frequent "motherly" kinds of interactions—the condition originally described by René Spitz as "hospitalism." It is not often seen now, but used to be more common in foundling homes and institutions where very few caretakers were responsible for too many infants, with no chance to do more than the essential impersonal tasks of baby care. There was no time for warm, loving interaction. A high percentage of such infants became listless, depressed, marasmic, and died. One cannot help but be reminded of the situation depicted in old ballads, romantic operas, and Victorian novels in which the pale heroine languished, pined away, and died of "unrequited love."

This discussion has covered some of the main features of the psychology of infanticide related to maltreatment, deaths due to acts of commission or omission, to abuse or neglect. It is a psychosocial problem of serious import; a conservative estimate is of two thousand deaths resulting from maltreatment each year in the United States. Such fatal outcomes represent only a small fraction of the enormous amount of irreparable physical and emotional damage caused by prevalent patterns of violent, unloving care of small children. The recent increasing interest in treatment and prevention of child abuse will gradually diminish this tragic "slaughter of the innocents." But the very nature of abuse and neglect leads to its endless repetition from generation to generation, which, coupled with the deep-seated historical roots of parental rights and cultural traditions of punishment, make it a formidable problem.

References

Adelson, L. "Slaughter of the Innocents." *New England J. of Med.* 264 (1961): 1345-49.

Bakan, David, *Slaughter of the Innocents: A Study of the Battered Child Phenomena.* San Francisco: Jossey-Bass Inc., 1971.

Cole, K. E., et al. "Women Who Kill." *Arch. Gen. Psychiat.* 19 (1968): 1-8.

Harder, T. "The Psychopathology of Infanticide." *Acta Psychiat. Scand.* 43 (1967): 196-245.

Kaplan, D., and Reich, R. "The Murdered Child and His Killers." *Amer. J. Psychiat.* 133 (1976): 809-815.

Meyerson, A. T. "Amnesia for Homicide ('Pedicide')." *Arch. Gen. Psychiat.* 14 (1966): 509-15.

Myers, S. A. "The Child Slayer." *Arch. Gen. Psychiat.* 17 (1968): 211-213.

Radbill, S. X. "A History of Child Abuse and Infanticide." In *The Battered Child.* Edited by Ray E. Helfer and C. Henry Kempe. Chicago: University of Chicago Press, 1968.

Resnick, P. J. "Child Murder by Parents: A Psychiatric Review of Filicide." *Amer. J. Psychiat.* 126 (1964): 325-334.

Spinetta, J. J., and Regler, D. "The Child-Abusing Parent: A Psychological Review." *Psychological Bulletin* 77 (1972): 296-301.

Steele, B., and Pollock, C. "A Psychiatric Study of Parents Who Abuse Infants and Small Children." In *The Battered Child.* Edited by Ray E. Helfer and C. Henry Kempe. Chicago: University of Chicago Press, 1968.

Steele, B. "Parental Abuse of Infants and Small Children." In *Parenthood: Its Psychology and Psychopathology.* Edited by E. James Anthony and Therese Benedek. Boston: Little, Brown, 1970.

Steele, B. "Violence Within the Family." In *Child Abuse and Neglect. The Family and the Community.* Edited by Ray E. Helfer and C. Henry Kempe. Cambridge, Mass.: Ballinger Publishing Co., 1976.

Peter Black

Killing and Allowing to Die

INTRODUCTION

In this paper, I wish to pay attention to the following kind of situation. A child is born with an illness that will certainly end in an early death but one that occurs unpredictably. For example, consider the child with leukemia before modern chemotherapy. The abnormality of his blood cells prevented him from killing invading bacteria; he was subjected to crisis after crisis when faced with the simplest of childhood infections. Ultimately the infections would become so overwhelming that the child would die from one particularly virulent one, but it was never altogether clear whether a given episode would be the last.

The question under consideration here is as follows. If a physician decides, at the outset of an infectious crisis, that he will withhold antibiotics, expecting the child to die, are his actions morally the same as giving the child enough intravenous sedative to kill him outright at that point? (He may, for example, feel that the pain and continued marginal, in-hospital, futile existence of the child warrant such management; for our purposes the parents will be presumed to agree with this completely.) Are the two courses of action morally identical?

Most of us would agree that giving a drug overdose is killing; many would argue that not treating an infection is "letting die" rather than "killing." The issue can therefore be restated: is "killing" in the sort of situation I have outlined the same as "letting die?" To use slightly different terminology: is there a morally important difference between so-called active euthanasia (the situation in which the agent does something to end life "actively") and passive euthanasia (the situation where the physician or other agent "lets nature take its course")?

Two points need clarification at the beginning. First, I am not suggesting that the physician should choose either to kill the child or let it die. The question is whether, once he has decided not to treat it as aggressively as he can, his actions are morally the same as giving it a known lethal drug. My inquiry is predicated on the conditional: if he decides not to treat vigorously expecting death to follow, is that the same as actively killing?

The second point is that the differences involved here are moral differences. Actions can be distinguished from each other in many ways; the question is whether the differences make them morally separate from each other. In a sense, this is a question about the moral values we wish to express. Some distinctions are not considered ethically relevant, the color of skin pigmentation being one contemporary example. The question here, therefore, is not so much whether some moral distinction between killing and letting die can possibly be made but rather what kind of values are expressed in the resulting moral code. Would we be willing to subscribe to the system that allows these distinctions?

There are at least three possible differences that have been suggested as being morally important in making a distinction between killing and letting die: (1) acting versus refraining; (2) causing death versus not causing death; (3) intending death versus not intending death. In the following pages I wish to discuss each briefly.

THREE POSSIBLE DISTINCTIONS

1. Acting, refraining, and responsibility

The first response a physician might make to the case presented in the first two paragraphs is: "The difference in the two situations is obvious: if I withhold antibiotics, I am carrying on a tradition in medicine of not using extraordinary means. If I give the child an overdose I am liable for murder in the courts of the state." This response has great importance; it recognizes that the physician has responsibilities to both society and patient; it points out that there does appear to be a barefaced difference between the two situations in medical tradition; and it implies that physicians as a group might feel there is important practical relevance in this difference.

There is not space in this paper to discuss the relation between principles and practicalities, between what ought to be done and what is done. It is true that our physician's answer may involve only "pragmatic" considerations, but the relationship of those to ethical rules cannot be ignored in a full discussion. Here I wish simply to point out that there is a weight of medical tradition separating killing from letting die. The question is whether an analysis of the two events demonstrates that such a distinction can be supported.

If our physician were pressed as to what further differences he could find, he might say: "In the situation of giving the overdose, I am actively doing something; in the other situation I am simply doing nothing." He might rely on a difference between acting and refraining as being morally significant.

It does seem that there is an involvement and immediacy in actively doing something that is not found in simply letting it occur. Surely, however, there are cases in which one is as culpable in *not* doing something as one ever could be in doing something.

Consider the following situation. Doctor X believes that a certain patient requiring a respirator should die. He is about to pull the respirator plug from the socket when a nurse trips on it and the respirator is disconnected. The nurse does not notice it, but Doctor X does and does nothing. The patient's breathing stops and he soon dies.

In Doctor Y's case, the nurse does not quite dislodge the plug. Y completes the job, removing it and watching as the patient dies.

Is there a difference between the situations? In the first, Dr. X might argue that he really did not do anything. Our moral evaluation, however, does not involve only what movements he made. It must also include whether he should have moved, what decisions he made, and what his responsibilities were for moving.[1] Both men have decided that the comatose patient should die. Do we feel that Doctor X, watching as the respirator plug is removed, is less culpable than the man who pulls the plug himself? (This assumes that X knows what is happening and is capable of replacing the plug.) Is there a morally relevant difference between leaving the plug out and pulling it out?

One way of approaching morally significant differences is to ask what is implied by their significance. If our system allowed only the agent himself to be held responsible for the results of an action, there would sometimes be patent injustice. The officer who orders his men to kill is an example; the Nuremberg war trials were uncompromising in their insistence that men be held responsible for the actions they assent to or instigate, as well as those they carry out themselves. By this criterion Doctor X is as guilty in leaving the plug out as Doctor Y is in removing it.

The cases seem different in this important way, however. In the "leaving the plug out" situation, there are many possible actions that might have been associated with the patient's death. The physician could have left the room, could in fact have been in another room all the time this was happening, or could have been honestly unaware that the plug had been pulled. The abundance of available moves makes it difficult to establish conclusively that the intention of allowing to die and the capability of preventing death were present at the same time. For the case of pulling the plug, the action seems to speak for itself. Retrospectively, it is more difficult to establish guilt in a letting die situation than a killing one. Prospectively, there is also greater difficulty. In prohibiting killing, we are proscribing one particular act or class of actions. If we were to try to prohibit letting die, the task would be harder because of the wide range of actions that could be construed as letting die. More constraints on our freedom of action are involved; in the pulling-the-plug situation, any action except replacing the plug is letting die. This is especially important in an ethical system such as ours in which minimal restrictions to personal freedom are desired. If we were to prohibit "letting die" generally, as we now prohibit "killing," we would require that an onlooker help a supposed victim. To give such help is of course desirable, but it is generally considered an act of grace rather than a moral requirement in our present system.[2]

In the medical example, however, considerations like these may not be relevant. There are certain instances in which we would naturally expect an onlooker to render aid, situations where it is easy to do so and the onlooker has a clear responsibility to maintain the well-being of the victim. These most parallel the medical case. There is a clear responsibility to maintain a patient's well-being involved in being a physician. This responsibility often overrides great difficulty in doing so; for a patient with a potentially good outcome physicians may expend immense time and talent in trying to "pull him through." The physician's action in the kind of problem we are postulating is a balance between two forces—his feeling of responsibility for the life of his patient, and the difficulty in maintaining that life. If he feels responsible enough for his patient, killing the patient and letting him die are equivalent for him. They can work both ways; he may decide that either action would be wrong, or he might feel that either action is justified. They are, in any case, ethically identical, for his involvement in the outcome is total.

The physician who does not feel responsible for his patient's survival at some point in his treatment might argue that at that point his job is not to try to thwart nature any longer. He might feel he should no longer try every means to keep his patient alive. In stopping treatment, however, he is not "letting die"; he is placing himself in the mass of men for whom no relation of responsibility for his patient's continued life can be drawn. A different responsibility—for example, easing suffering— may then become his major concern. Not treating is then not a consignment to inevitable death; it is denying one's responsibility for supporting the patient's life any longer. One distinction between acting and refraining develops as a difference in responsibilities; on the one hand, an abnegation of the responsibility to keep alive; on the other, a refusal of the responsibility to kill.

There are two other ways of looking at the difference between killing and letting die that may also be morally relevant in certain circumstances. They are from the viewpoints of causation and intentions.

2. Causing and not causing

A physician confronted with our opening situation might argue the following: "If I simply do not treat this child's infection, the cause of his death is his leukemia or sepsis. If I give him an overdose of medication, my action is the cause of his death. Therefore there is a difference between killing and letting die that is morally important."

A first response to this might be to ask whether death in either case is bad. We might argue that death for this child is a blessing, and that, therefore, there is no greater evil associated with killing than with letting die.

However, if we leave the goodness of his death open to question, there is still a comment to be made about causation in this context. Naming the cause of death continues to be a problem in medicine. In most instances, the ultimate cause is cardiac arrest, which may be preceded by many other events. These can range from strangulation to sudden cardiac arrhythmias to whatever it is that cancer does to cause death. Physicians do not generally say the cause of death is cardiac arrest, however. On the death certificate this is called the mechanism of death. The cause appears to be something more difficult to define. Without developing the idea in detail, I would suggest that the "cause" of death is the event that made a difference in what would have been the predicted outcome. It is the item responsible for a change in a patient's course.[3] As such, it is singled out to fit the explanatory scheme we are using. When a man has increasing difficulty breathing because of fluid build-up in the lung, the cause of death is felt to be the disease producing a heart too weak to pump all his blood. There may be several other factors involved as well that contribute to his death, but the primary one is the one that seems to explain the change in the usual course of his life.

Can an omission—a negative action—be considered a cause? It seems clear that it should be. When a man lapsing into insulin coma needs only sugar to prevent ultimate death, deliberate failure to provide that sugar can certainly be considered part of the cause of his death.

There is a peculiarity about assigning causes that must be mentioned, however. When I fail to give sugar to a man I know is in insulin coma, my omission contributes to his death. It is, however, his diabetes that killed him. My omission is not considered the major cause of his death, even though without it he may have survived. This is even more true in the case of withholding antibiotics from a leukemic child. The cause of his death is leukemia with infection, not a lack of antibiotics.

If I proceed to give him an overdose of barbiturates, the situation is quite different. Here the cause of death is my drug. Even though I argue that the reason for my giving the drug is his leukemia, this does not change the fact that his death was caused by my actions.

The reason for this difference seems to be partly the unpredictability of medical events. If we knew absolutely that an antibiotic would cure the child and that not giving it would kill him, my refusal to treat could more clearly be seen as causative. Nature, however, is less predictable than this; my act of not treating may leave several outcomes possible. Thus, at best, my refusal to treat becomes one of many causes in his death.

It is perhaps the difference between being one of many causes and

91

being the major cause that allows a moral distinction to be made between killing and letting die on the basis of causing and not causing death. In the killing case, the major cause is the action that led to death. In the letting-die case, the inaction that led to death is more clearly seen as one of many circumstances necessary to result in death.

3. Intention

The final issue is whether intention can be used as a distinguishing feature between killing and letting die. Could a physician say in facing the infected leukemic child: "If I do not give him the antibiotic, I am not intending his death; I am just practicing medicine in a certain way. If I give him an overdose deliberately, however, I must be intending his death directly."

An initial question involves what the physician expects in the situation we have hypothesized. We are excluding ignorance as a reason for not giving antibiotics, or suspected allergy to the antibiotic, or a belief that the child has a better chance of living without them. We are assuming that the physician is withholding medication with the expectation that the child will die following his inaction.

Does he then intend the child's death? If he does intend it, is he therefore guilty if it occurs and is considered a bad outcome?

These questions require more space than this discussion will permit. They have been approached briefly in contemporary literature pertaining to this problem. They lead into the topic of the double effect, which has had wide theological and philosophical study.[4] Briefly, one might argue that the death of a patient following withholding of treatment is foreseen but not intended primarily. The primary intention may be to relieve suffering or to stop useless treatment. Death is then an expected but not direct goal of stopping treatment. In giving a lethal drug, on the other hand, the outcome of death must be seen as a more direct goal.

Another way of looking at this is to suggest that in withholding treatment certain other considerations are primary, and death is acceptable as a byproduct of those. Again, relieving suffering may be the major "other" consideration, but so may maintaining one's role as a professional or obeying the laws of the society. Actions which allow these and result in death may be more morally acceptable than those which transgress them by intending death as a primary action.

This is a complicated area in moral reasoning, and this paper will just suggest that it may contain a third relevant difference between killing and letting die. More detailed analysis is necessary before such a claim can be accepted.

SUMMARY AND CONCLUSIONS

This discussion began with a case in which some writers would consider killing and letting die morally equivalent. It involved withholding antibiotics from a child who would be helped only temporarily by them. It introduced the claim that withholding was the same action morally as killing the child outright, and asked what possible rejoinders could be produced to this claim.

Three possible differences between the two actions have been proposed. The first was that withholding was different than killing because it was refraining, not acting. This had two implications: first, the possible outcomes were thereby left more open; second, it allowed the agent to continue to be responsible for something to benefit the patient, rather than simply for killing him. It was seen as denial of the responsibility for maintaining life to withhold treatment, but not as an undertaking of a responsibility to kill.

The second difference was based on causal relationships. In the case of letting die, the withholding of antibiotics is one of several events implicated in the patient's death. In killing, the human action is more likely to be seen as the major causal event.

The third proposed distinction was based on intentions. In the withholding-of-treatment situation, the intention of letting die might be seen as a secondary one justified by a wish to help or a wish to be a good physician. It was therefore different than the situation where death is a primary goal. This possibility was not developed fully.

These three kinds of distinction may all be possible ways of arguing that killing is different than letting die. They involve an analysis of the two actions. The question remains whether we as a society would want to maintain the distinctions that can be made using these analyses.

This is a question that cannot be answered here. The primary purpose of this paper is to ask whether a difference between killing and let-

PETER BLACK

ting die can be supported; that is, whether there are any moral viewpoints that allow such a distinction. Intention, causation, and acting-
refraining have been proposed as three such viewpoints. One might ask
the following questions, however. Should our society have a moral system in which intentions are not necessarily considered the same as expected outcomes, or where a so-called "primary intention" can outweigh
a "secondary" one? Are we justified in a usage of causal notions that
says withholding a life-saving antibiotic is not causing death in the same
way that giving a lethal drug is? Is it defensible to argue that leaving
many possibilities open by refraining from acting is morally better than
doing a particular action?

These are questions that must be answered by whatever methods
moral issues are resolved for a particular group or individual. It is worth
pointing out, however, the importance of the physician's role and responsibility in such a decision. There are at least two views of his role in
which the physician might feel that killing and letting die are morally
equivalent. The first is the view that life must be preserved at all costs.
With this outlook, killing and letting die are both morally unacceptable,
but are equally so. The other is the outlook that life and death decisions
for his patients are entirely in a physician's power to carry out. In this situation, too, killing and letting die will be morally equivalent, but will
both be morally acceptable. From this viewpoint, for example, the imperative to relieve suffering might allow killing as legitimately as it does
letting die.

Suppose, however, a physician thinks that life should be preserved
but not at all costs, and that deliberate causation of death by a direct act
is a very serious matter morally. It may then be important to him to
decide whether there are situations in which letting die is morally permissible but killing is not. The first step in deciding this seems to be
working out what possible differences might be developed between those
two situations. This paper has attempted to begin such a "working out."
From it may be developed the moral justifications for the differences
suggested embryonically here.

Notes

1. James Rachels has presented a similar case in "Active and Passive Euthanasia," *New
England Journal of Medicine* 292 (January 9, 1975): 78-80. Smith and Jones both wish to

94

drown a nephew. Smith does so; Jones watches as his nephew slips and falls in the bathtub, dying without Jones's help. Rachels claims that the mere fact of acting versus refraining makes no difference.

2. P. J. Fitzgerald has developed this concept in "Acting and Refraining," *Analysis* 27: 133-139. The place of role considerations and responsibility is best presented in John Casey's long essay, "Actions and Consequences," in *Morality and Moral Reasoning*, ed. J. Casey (London: Methuen, 1971).

3. This formulation of causation is best expressed in H. L. A. Hart and A. M. Honoré, *Causation in the Law* (Clarendon: Oxford University Press, 1959).

4. Richard McCormick has developed a modern theological view of this doctrine in "Ambiguity and Moral Choice," the Marquette lectures, 1971.

Philippa Foot has perhaps the best-known philosophical restatement of the doctrine in "The Problem of Abortion and the Doctrine of the Double Effect," reprinted in James Rachels, ed., *Moral Problems: A Collection of Philosophical Essays*, 2nd ed. (New York: Harper and Row, 1975).

Raymond S. Duff

Deciding the Care of Defective Infants

Since entering medicine twenty-nine years ago, the author and probably a growing number of colleagues and citizens have been forced to acknowledge that our attitudes and practices regarding who shall live or die and how must be revised if we truly care about people.[1] Those who have reported their feelings and hopes in tragic situations eventually reach this conclusion on humanitarian grounds and commonly reject dogmas contending otherwise. The situation of defective infants examined in this paper illustrates some of the problems.

In earlier centuries, 10 to 20 percent of infants commonly died in the first month of life, and up to 50 percent or more died before one year of age. People appeared to be resigned to these high death rates, and infanticide, especially of defective infants, was condoned. But things have changed. Improved nutrition and housing, advances in medicine, and possibly other factors were associated with a sharp decline in mortality rates. By 1915, only 10 percent of infants died in the United States in the first year of life. The corresponding figure for 1975 was 1.6 percent.[2] With the development of collaborative obstetric, pediatric, anesthesia, and other services in providing perinatal care, these rates likely will decline further.[3] While some infants are "allowed" to die, this is viewed as a failure, and active infanticide, if it exists at all, is hidden. Fortunately in this success story, lower mortality rates have been associated with

96

higher quality of life among the survivors.

However, not all is well. While 90–95 percent of fetuses with the most severe abnormalities are discarded by spontaneous abortion or stillbirth,[4] the remainder often have problems beyond hope of correction. Prematurity without abnormality of body structure commonly involves numerous respiratory, nutritional, infectious, and other problems. The results of treating an individual infant with major anomalies or severe prematurity often cannot be predicted accurately. They may include a reasonably healthy infant, one impaired in varying degrees, or death. Medical technology complicates the prognosis because it may harm babies as well as help them. Life-saving use of oxygen may damage the lungs or blind the eyes. Antibiotics may save the lives of some infants but their brains sometimes have been damaged by treatment. Medical technology is necessarily intrusive. It commonly hurts, often harms, and can be cruel. Yet it may provide minimal or no benefits in some situations.

Baby Girl U illustrates these problems. Apparently in good health at birth, she developed symptoms of bowel obstruction (from a malformation) at thirty-four hours of age. At surgery, most of her necrotic bowel was removed to save her life. Intravenous nutrition was given in hope of eventual adequate bowel function. However, such substitutions commonly have complications as happened in this case, and they cannot be effective in the long run. By four months of age, intravenous support was increasingly problematic and the bowel was not functioning. While the baby was given every advantage of treatment, she had been put through several operations and had endured constant manipulations and treatments.

At two days of age, this baby's chances of long-term survival were estimated to be very low (perhaps less than one in ten thousand). Her suffering had been fully anticipated. Should we (family and health professionals) have chosen to treat her at all? If not, should we have let her cruel disease kill her or should we ease her into death, perhaps by killing her in a more kindly way? Should we continue treatment now despite apparent hopelessness? If so, how can we justify our cruelty? If not, should we kill her gently, as some suggested when she was two days of age? Apart from any influence for better or worse of this child's tragic plight upon the family and society, many reasonable, caring persons from the family and the hospital staff considered that killing this child at any time after two days of age was potentially less tragic than treating her as we did.

RAYMOND S. DUFF

Families invariably are affected by illness of a member. The U family, for example, mobilized its resources and seemed strengthened at first. However, family life deteriorated under psychological and financial stresses after the first month of the baby's life. This family, as Haggerty suggested for others,[5] had overestimated and overcommitted its financial and other resources. This was done because of their concerns and hopes for their baby and because they mistook the doctor's *enthusiasm* to treat the baby for *optimism* about outcome. They came to regret the choice to treat their baby because they felt that was cruel to her and damaging to the family. They came to believe an early death would have been better and rejected further life-sustaining treatment. The baby died slowly of dehydration and starvation. The parents, nurses, and doctors felt there should have been a better way of caring.

Soon after the baby's death, a nurse who had cared for her had a dream. In this, she was holding her own defective baby in her left arm as he died. In her right hand, she held a gun aimed at the doctors and nurses to prevent them from applying inappropriate treatment. After telling us about this dream, she added, "it's so sad that conditions here are sometimes such that I have to dream like that."

Decisions to treat Baby Girl U have implications for society. Knowledge possibly helpful to others in the future was gained by trying to correct her problems. The hospital, the companies that supply materials, and those who work in the hospital received income from that vast sum ($140 billion per year and rising) allocated for health resources in the United States. In addition to what the U family paid, other citizens through insurance premiums or taxes paid $43 thousand. Some citizens paid in other ways. Since Baby Girl U required much intensive care, some persons believed other sick infants and well infants in the same hospital often were neglected during her hospital stay. Since such concerns may be multiplied by thousands across the land, it is appropriate to ask to what extent the extremely high cost of health care results from doing harmful things to people.

Considering the decline in infant mortality rates from some 50 percent to 1.6 percent in the last few centuries, and in light of continuing natural selection by prematurity and congenital anomalies, it is obvious that dramatic, additional lowering of mortality rates for severely defective infants is impossible, and that further reductions of mortality can be achieved only by relatively large expenditures of money and other forms of human energy. Beyond some point, this simply will not be done. The

98

reason is plain: there are competing values that may be of equal or greater importance. Other persons also live. They have some power and no doubt will use it. Presumably they should, unless one accepts the notion that caring for the sick or deformed is the only significant value in life. But this tyranny of the sick over the well may be as objectionable as tyranny of the well over the sick.

Awareness of these social issues was reflected by a pediatrician who wrote in a recent text on neonatology: "How does one answer a kindly congressman in a House appropriations subcommittee, constrained by the limits of the federal budget-making process, when he wants to know whether one should save very low-birth-weight infants, even if it should prove there is a reduction in incidence of moderate and severe handicap from 85 to 50 percent?"[6] Almost everyone is partial to the development and use of medical technology. But in view of the consequences of patient care decisions for infants, families, and society, the reasoning in this paper clearly leads to a policy of *selected* application. In fact, practices consistent with this policy exist. However, since they often are not acknowledged, they are not discussed, and decisions may be taken with careless regard for values. Indeed, it is possible that more killing is now done by subterfuge than would be done if there were freedom to choose openly. It is likely, however, that more harm is currently done by compulsory living.

The public should know that it is often misled by its own pressing desire for hope and by well-meaning though perhaps exploiting professionals. Gellis, an internationally known pediatrician, author, and editor, acknowledges this dilemma in his complaint that most results of using medical technology have been reported by those who provided the care. They may be biased (for understandable reasons) so as to hide some dismal results. He reviewed two recent, conflicting reports and asked, "How much are we accomplishing by our gadgetry?"[7]

To care for people as Mayeroff, for example, views caring,[8] the following options should be available. As far as technology is developed and useful, persons may choose to apply it even if the cost is high and suffering great. Or, holding to another order of values, they may reject technology and "let nature take its course." Or, since some persons may find that both treatment and the disease are more cruel than death, they may kill. Of course, before death any decision for care may be changed as conditions indicate. Essential procedures in deciding care involve careful evaluation of biological situations, meticulous review of personal and family values, truth telling, and examination of expected consequences for all potential choices. As in other aspects of caring, patients (when able), families, and their professional advisors in that order of decisional power should choose. In this decentralized model for deciding care, there is no chance for a holocaust. But since poor choices no doubt may be made from time to time, great care must be taken to control misguided altruism on the one hand and selfishness on the other.

Some may argue that patients, families, and health professionals are incapable of analyzing problems and deciding care in this fashion. The author and almost all families he has seen find otherwise.[9] Most persons, despite grief, will cope with tragic realities when these are understood. Surely, puzzling out the decisions for care will be untidy. But that is one of the features of high quality decision making.[10] What is most needed now is some freedom to exercise virtue even though a few mistakes will be made. If caring is to be optimal, coercive living like coercive dying has no place among our choices. The decision to be or not to be is liberating because some measure of control is maintained in the face of death and apparent helplessness.

If the above constitutes a prudent approach to some vexing issues in human affairs, the medical profession and the public have a lot of explaining to do and risks to take, because it is unlikely that courts or legislatures will take initiative to reform. There may be a constitutional issue in all this. Current laws evidently presume guilt of persons in deciding on death or on many conditions of dying *before* acts are taken. That seems inconsistent with the notion of presuming innocence until proven guilty. However, it appears the climate in the legislatures will have to change greatly if we are to get anywhere with this issue there. Ironically, the attempt in California probably had the opposite result of what was desired. The recently passed euthanasia law probably makes it more difficult than ever to die in that state.[11]

Recently, several family practitioners have told the author that the problem of choosing death and acting accordingly exists chiefly in institutions. There, in a semipublic place, as contrasted to the homes of citizens, a pleasant-appearing and comfortable morality must prevail. Choices are restricted by the need to avoid controversy and to live within perhaps the most restricted interpretation of the law. In addition, in our teaching hospitals where student professionals are taught habits which may endure for a lifetime, patients subtilely are compelled by what one spokesman called the "service thermostat" to accept "treatment" decisions representing a combination of interests: patient care, teaching, and research. In these same institutions, the patients often come from poor families, so that resistance to oppressive treatment may be minimal.[12]

Perhaps Manning is correct when he writes, "the better course at this time would appear to be to address the topic in low key, to bring about gradual public education of the matter, and, for the time being, to leave to informal processes the slow development of commonly understood standards within the medical profession."[13] But that does not comfort those in the present who are trapped in the tyranny of laggardly laws.[14]

Notes

1. Albert R. Jonsen and Michael J. Garland, eds., *Ethics of Newborn Intensive Care* (Berkeley, Calif.: Institute of Governmental Studies, 1976).

2. Myron E. Wegman, "Annual Summary of Vital Statistics—1975," *Pediatrics* 58 (1976): 793-799.

3. P. M. Fitzhardinge, K. Pape, et al., "Mechanical Ventilation of Infants Less Than 1501 gm Birth Weight: Health, Growth, and Neurologic Sequelae," *Journal of Pediatrics* 88 (1976): 531-541.

4. J. L. Hamerton, N. Canning, et al., "Cytogenetic Survey of 14,069 Newborn Infants," *Clinical Genetics* 8 (1975): 223-243.

5. Robert J. Haggerty, Klaus J. Roghmann, and Ivan B. Pless, *Child Health and the Community* (New York: John Wiley and Sons, 1975), pp. 41-66.

6. Gordon B. Avery, ed., *Neonatology, Pathophysiology and Management of the Newborn* (Philadelphia: J. B. Lippincott, 1975), p. 8.

7. Sidney S. Gellis, *The Year Book of Pediatrics* (Chicago: Year Book Medical Publishers, 1976), p. 23.

8. Milton Mayeroff, *On Caring* (New York: Harper and Row, 1971).

9. R. S. Duff, "On Deciding the Use of the Family Commons," *Birth Defects: Original Article Series* 12: 73-84, The National Foundation, 1976.

10. David Braybrooke and Charles E. Lindblom, *A Strategy of Decision* (New York: The Free Press, 1970).

11. Michael Garland, "Politics, Legislation, and Natural Death," *Hastings Center Report* 6 (1976): 5-6.

12. R. S. Duff, "Patient Care, the Poor, and Medical Education," *Poverty and Health: A Sociological Analysis*, ed. John Kosa and Irving Zola (Cambridge, Mass.: Harvard University Press, 1975), pp. 335-350.

13. Bayless Manning, "Legal and Policy Issues in the Allocation of Death," *The Dying Patient*, ed. Orville G. Brimm, Jr. et al. (New York: Russell Sage Foundation, 1970), p. 270.

14. Daniel Maguire, *Death by Choice* (Garden City, N.Y.: Doubleday and Company, 1974).

Anthony Shaw

Who Should Die
and Who Should Decide?

I had the good fortune back in 1968 to spend several months with Project HOPE in Ceylon (now Sri Lanka). During my brief tenure as visiting pediatric surgeon to the Lady Ridgeway Children's Hospital in Colombo, I assisted at an operation on a newborn infant with gastroschisis, a condition in which the entire intestinal tract is exposed through a hole in the infant's navel—a catastrophic problem requiring the most urgent and sophisticated surgical management. Although the operation was performed meticulously, the baby died several hours later because of absence of the supportive equipment and personnel required in the surgical "follow-through." The next day one of the young hospital residents remarked to me "that was an interesting academic exercise."[1]

In the well-staffed and superbly equipped medical centers of the United States, however, the predictable success of such operations on newborn infants with complex congenital malformations is widely regarded as among the major accomplishments of Western medicine. Advances in diagnostic, surgical, and anesthetic techniques have enabled pediatric surgeons like myself to correct many kinds of congenital defects that were pathological curiosities only a few years ago. Newborn intensive care nurseries, staffed by physicians specializing in neonatal medicine (neonatologists), and by highly trained intensive care nurse specialists who utilize the latest models of vital sign monitoring equipment, blood oxygen and pH analyzers, miniature respirators, and other life support systems assure that most of our little patients will recover and go home—not become merely "an interesting academic exercise."

By establishing and supporting such expensive facilities for tiny, premature, desperately ill, and severely malformed infants on regional bases through combinations of tax dollars, national and community philanthropies, and financial sleight-of-hand by hospital administrators; by developing efficient transport mechanisms to guarantee their safe arrival —networks of intensive care units on wheels, ambulance helicopters, Lear jets—society seems to have made a decision to go all out to rescue all newborn life. Whether such a trend has stemmed from a genuine concern for the survival and welfare of our newest and most vulnerable citizens, from a national and regional embarrassment at our relatively high ranking among Western nations in neonatal mortality, or from medical and industrial imperatives to apply our latest technology as it develops (or from all three), society, by creating the intensive care nursery and its support and feeder mechanisms, seems to have expressed a commitment to salvaging all distressed human newborn life.

Few of the doctors and nurses who work in the exciting and generally rewarding environment of intensive care nurseries are critical of the basic philosophy underlying their establishment, and fewer still would wish to curtail the public enthusiasm with which they are currently supported; and yet, in spite of the fact that the ICNs are dedicated to newborn survival, many recent articles (including some by this author) document circumstances under which infants, on reaching the supposed sanctuary of the intensive care nursery, are deliberately being allowed to die by those very individuals traditionally committed to the welfare of babies—physicians and parents. This seeming inconsistency between action and intent results from the success of the intensive care nursery in keeping babies alive, a success that in turn has raised ethical and moral dilemmas more complex than some of the medical problems for which the units were designed.

The first question in a recent national survey of pediatricians and pediatric surgeons asked: "Do you believe that the life of each and every newborn infant should be saved if it is within our ability to do so?"[2]

Eighty-two percent of the 447 respondents replied "No." Analysis of the correlation between responses to this question and religious faiths of the respondents reveal that a large majority of physicians in each major religious group (Protestant, Catholic, Jewish) as well as of those professing no formal faith does not feel morally obligated to attempt salvage of every newborn human life. (That this belief translates into practice is amply documented in articles by such practicing physicians as Duff,[3] Girvan and Stephens,[4] and Lorber.[5]) Duff, who heads the intensive care nursery at Yale-New Haven Hospital, reported 299 deaths in his unit during 1970–1972. Forty-three of these deaths (14 percent) resulted from withdrawing or withholding treatment. Girvan and Stephens, in an article describing the surgical management of intestinal obstruction in newborns, reported that of a group of fifty babies who also had Down's syndrome (mongolism), the parents of twenty-seven refused surgery after a ". . . careful explanation of the alternatives." Lorber, a British pediatrician and neurologist, has widely published his criteria for choosing which infants with spina bifida cystica (meningomyelocele) should be treated. (His selective nontreatment results in early death of those children born with the most severe manifestations of this complex malformation.)

What circumstances cause a majority of pediatric surgeons and of chairmen of university departments of pediatrics to agree that some babies whose lives could be prolonged should be allowed to die? In the survey the question was put as follows: "If you agree under certain circumstances it is permissable to allow certain severely damaged infants to die by withholding surgical treatment, select the criteria for making such a decision in order of priority."

"Potential quality of life of the infant" was chosen to head the list of the five possible choices; "possible adverse effects on the infant's family" came in second while "cost to society" ran a distant fifth. ("Infant's probable IQ" and "parents' willingness to raise the child at home" were third and fourth respectively.)

What, from the *infant's* point of view, could justify letting it die? A qualitatively meaningless life? A life of vegetative, noncognitive existence, or one doomed to early extinction, or a life of constant frustration or pain? Many writers have tried, in recent years, to supply a definition of "meaningful" that might justify the efforts we make on behalf of the lives of impaired newborns—or conversely—justify letting go of a life lacking this quality of "meaningfulness."

Some, like McCormick,[6] believe the essence of a "meaningful life" is an ability to form relationships. Others, agreeing with Fletcher,[7] would define it in terms of quantitative indicators of humanhood or personhood. Reich has viewed it as the ability to say "Yes" to life.[8] Although.

philosophers may debate the question of whether there is such a thing as a life not worth living, many physicians, including myself, agree that there are such lives and that we, through our applied technology, have perpetuated many of them along with the much larger number of "worthwhile" lives we save.[9] These are not the kinds of standards scientifically trained physicians like, but science has not been very helpful here either. (Scientists are having a hard enough time defining what they mean by the term "life" itself, let alone a "meaningful" one.)

Whether or not a consensus is reached on the meaning of "meaningful," decisions to treat or not to treat severely impaired newborns are clearly being made by physicians and parents on considerations based on an estimate of *quality of life.* If decisions to treat or not to treat are indeed based on quality of life calculations, it might be possible to identify the factors determining quality of life, place them within the context of a mathematical formula, and thereby produce a rough estimate of the potential quality of life of an individual. One formula which expresses the inclination of many physicians to equate quality of life with physical or mental characteristics could read QL = NE where QL represents the quality of life and NE represents the natural endowment, physical and mental, of the individual under consideration.[10]

If we apply this formula to a newborn infant whose life will be of short duration despite our best efforts and whose prognosis for cognitive existence during that span is nil, we would assess that infant's NE at zero. The infant's QL would therefore also equal zero.

Not surprisingly then, the physicians responding to our survey were almost unanimous in assenting to the withholding of lifesaving surgical procedures for infants with anencephaly or 13-15 trisomy, conditions predictably in this zero NE catagory.[11]

However, for newborns with lesser degrees of impairment (Down's syndrome, multiple limb deformities, meningomyelocele), the consensus for nontreatment declines as estimates of NE of infants rise. Moreover, it is clear that for infants whose NE is greater than zero, additional factors may add to or subtract from the QL. These factors are the familial and societal influences that affect an infant's QL in either a positive or negative manner. Thus a better approximation of potential quality of life is made possible by expanding the above formula as follows:

QL = NE × (H + S), where H and S represent the contributions *to* the infant under consideration from home (family) and society respectively.

Clearly if the family of a baby with a Down's syndrome refused to care for it, and society's sole contribution is a crowded, filthy, understaffed warehouse, that infant's quality of life equals zero (NE $\times$ (0+0) = 0) just as surely as if it had been born an anencephalic.

It is not surprising then that the degree of effort made by many physicians on behalf of some defective newborns is directly related to the willingness of families and/or communities to provide sufficient resources and support to compensate for these infants' deficient NE. If, as Robert Louis Stevenson wrote, "Life is not a matter of holding good cards, but of playing a poor hand well," the impaired individual needs that help from H and S if he is to play his hand at all.

There are practical difficulties in basing treatment versus nontreatment decisions on meaningfulness or other quality of life criteria. Oftentimes the focus of the discussion on treatment decisions becomes blurred because it is unclear which life is at issue. This may occur during a medical conference (one in which assessment of QL is critical to the outcome) where the focus of the discussion can shift imperceptibly from the potential quality of life of the impaired infant to that of his parents, siblings, or even to that of society at large. Although many of the factors determining the quality of life of the child may also determine the quality of life of his family members, such factors often affect them differently; therefore, if one wishes to examine the effects of alternative courses of action on the quality of life of family and child, it is important not to lose sight of whose quality of life is being examined at each step in the decision-making process. Thinking in terms of the formula format may help prevent such confusion. For example, if we are considering the potential quality of life of a newborn infant with Down's syndrome, factors dealing with the willingness of his parents to nurture him, to support him at home, to love him, to provide resources for special training and education belong in a calculation of QL_{baby}. Factors such as the contributions the infant will make to the understanding and maturing of his siblings, the extent to which he will reinforce the egos of other family members, the financial and emotional burden he will place on his parents belong in a calculation of QL_{family}.[12]

To what extent should the impact of a defective infant on the well-being of his family be a factor in treatment versus nontreatment decisions? The respondents to our survey gave this consideration second priority to that of "potential quality of life of the infant." The survey indicated that many physicians would acquiesce in parents' wishes not to treat their defective infants because of negative effects on the QL of the family stemming from such factors as marital or emotional instability, inadequate financial resources, potential adverse effects on siblings, and so on.

However, the survey made it clear that physicians differ considerably among themselves in their perceptions of the quality of life associated with conditions of moderate severity such as Down's syndrome and also differ greatly in their impressions of the extent to which such impaired infants adversely affect their families.

Finally while the "cost to society" criterion for life and death decision making was ranked lowest by the survey respondents, it is of major significance and makes its influence felt wherever the political process determines priorities in the allocation of medical resources. Which babies we save and who decides which ones will be saved is often determined by such political and economic considerations as those referred to in my opening paragraphs with respect to the funding and staffing of intensive care nurseries.[13]

Looking to the future, the resolution of such issues as life and death decision making may depend on the relative strengths of opposing societal forces, some of which may be identified at present.

Examples of forces which have tended to restrict parental and physician discretionary decision making are as follows:

Anti-abortion lobbying groups (If the vocal and well-organized "right to life" forces are successful in their efforts to turn back the clock on abortion, it will again be illegal to abort a fetus simply because a diagnostic amniocentesis has proved it is irreparably impaired. It would seem unlikely, in such a climate, that parents and physicians will continue to be granted the discretion society now tacitly allows them to occasionally make the terribly difficult decision not to treat a newborn baby.);

Legislation requiring availability and utilization of life-support measures for products of abortions or miscarriages;

Provision of financial incentives for foster care or adoption of impaired babies;

Court decisions in which considerations of quality of life are rejected (Notably in the well-publicized cases of Baby Houle and Karen Ann Quinlan in which Judges Roberts[14] and Muir[15] respectively rejected quality of life considerations in ordering continuing life-sustaining treatment for severely damaged individuals whose parents opposed such efforts.);

Political pressure to minimize the perinatal death rate;

Fear of the slippery slope ("If we do not do all we can to save the severely brain-damaged newborn with congenital heart disease and intestinal obstruction, it won't be long before we start killing off the old people and Jews.");

Child abuse and neglect laws (Most such legislation defines as "medical neglect" the failure of parents to provide "necessary medical care" for their children and threatens physicians with prosecution for failure to report such "neglect.");

Criminal statutes. (Robertson[16] has pointed out a wide range of laws that may be invoked, although they have not been as yet, by public prosecutors to bring charges ranging from misdemeanor to conspiracy to homicide against physicians who allow severely impaired infants to die.)

Examples of societal forces which tend to broaden parental and professional discretion include:

Enactment of state "Death with Dignity" or "Natural Death" laws (Such laws reflect a widely held belief that if, at some point, life quality deteriorates to such a low level that death becomes a preferable alternative, this kind of legislation may be necessary to prevent the artificial prolongation of a terminal state.);

Application of cost-benefit analysis to medical resource allocation (With realization that the earth's resources are limited and that with the enormous increases in the cost of medical care, especially in such areas as chronic disease and intensive care of adults and infants, continuing efforts to provide the fruits of medical knowledge and technology to everyone will clearly have to be modified by cost-benefit analyses of the whole spectrum of human needs.);[17]

Increasing acceptance by courts of a definition of death that equates death of the individual with death of the brain (Such a definition of death reflects the perception that the brain, not the heart or lungs, is central to our concept of meaningful human life—a concept that is in opposition to the idea that as long as any human cells are biologically functioning, the body in which they are housed must still be considered a living human being to be sustained at any cost.);

Increasing acceptability of nonutilization of extraordinary means to prolong lives of the critically ill. (In his introduction of "ordinary means" to the treatment versus nontreatment dialogue, Pope Pius XII supplied physicians with a practical and humane semantic device for resolving some of their dilemmas.)

Perhaps future breakthroughs in the treatment of afflictions of the central nervous system and widespread acceptance of family planning, birth control, and selective abortion may make most of our current ethical problems in the newborn nursery obsolete. For the present, however, so long as discretionary decision making in the matter of defective newborns is tolerated by society, I believe, as do most of my colleagues,[18] that the most humane manner for resolving these issues is on a case by case basis, whereby parents and physicians reach a decision that reflects primarily a concern for the quality of that newborn life.

Notes

1. The operation on some infants with life-threatening birth defects may be the easiest, briefest, and least expensive aspect of the management of a complex malformation. Intensive postoperative management of derangements of gastrointestinal, respiratory, and cardiovascular systems, often complicated by organ immaturity in premature infants, may go on for weeks or months.

2. Anthony Shaw, J. G. Randolph, and B. Manard, "Ethical Issues in Pediatric Surgery: A National Survey of Pediatricians and Pediatric Surgeons," *Pediatrics* 60 (Suppl.): 588-599, 1977.

The survey questionnaire was sent to all members of the Surgical Section of the American Academy of Pediatrics, all Chairmen of Departments of Pediatrics, and all Chiefs of Divisions of Genetics and Neonatology within Departments of Pediatrics.

3. R. S. Duff and A. G. M. Campbell, "Moral and Ethical Dilemmas in the Special Care Nursery," *New England Journal of Medicine* 289 (1973): 890-894.

4. D. P. Girvan and C. A. Stephens, "Congenital Intrinsic Duodenal Obstruction," *Journal of Pediatric Surg.* 9 (1974): 833-839.

5. J. Lorber, "Results of Treatment of Myelomeningocele: An Analysis of 524 Unselected Cases with Special Reference to Possible Selection for Treatment," *Develop. Med. Child. Neurol.* 13 (1971): 279.

6. R. A. McCormick, "To Save or Let Die: The Dilemma of Modern Medicine," *JAMA* 229 (1974): 172-176.

7. J. Fletcher, "Indicators of Humanhood: A Tentative Profile of Man," *The Hastings Center Report* 2 (1972): 1-4.

8. W. T. Reich, "Quality of Life: Ethical Considerations in the Newborn Child," (Paper presented at a conference on spina bifida and ethics, "Decisionmaking and the Defective Newborn," held at Skytop, Pennsylvania, May 4-7, 1975).

9. ". . . some infants are saved from early death only for an existence which few people would consider worth living" (A. R. Jonsen, R. H. Phibbs, W. H. Tooley, and M. J. Garland, "Critical Issues in Newborn Intensive Care: A Conference Report and Policy Proposal," *Pediatrics* 55 [1975]: 756-768).

This article by Jonsen et al. provides the best analysis of the clinical-ethical dilemmas raised by neonatal intensive care to date, and represents one of the few efforts to develop guidelines, understandable and potentially helpful, to physicians. The authors are sympathetic to the needs of both the impaired newborns and their families.

10. This formula and the subsequent one were initially conceived and presented by the author in a paper, "Ethics of Proxy Consent," at a conference, "Decisionmaking and the Defective Newborn," chaired by Dr. Chester Swinyard at Skytop, Pennsylvania, May 4-7, 1975.

11. Solid medical expertise is fundamental to the consideration of nontreatment options which are based on estimates of NE. As a result of improved diagnostic capabilities (e.g.,

chromosome and enzyme analysis) the poor prognosis of certain congenital conditions can be accurately predicted and extraordinary efforts on behalf of such infants appropriately withdrawn. Conversely, improved life support systems allow us to keep advancing our therapeutic frontiers to reverse the previously irreversible, allowing us to save, for example, smaller and smaller premature infants and babies with less and less intestine (at great cost, of course), making it difficult to predict on the basis of past experience that a particular infant will not survive with current efforts. Thus, while for some categories of infants NE becomes easier to predict, for others (such as small prematures, infants with severe pulmonary damage, and infants with short bowel syndrome) it may become more difficult.

12. The QL of a child, whether impaired or not, often bears an inverse relationship to that of his parents, in that the parents' contribution of time and treasure, which enhance the quality of life of the child, reduces those resources that they might use for enhancement of their own lives. (When the same considerations are extended to society we are talking about cost-benefit analysis.) Such a conflict lies at the heart of making a decision with respect to institutionalizing a retarded child, for example. This is well-illustrated in *Wyatt* versus *Stickney*, Amici Briefs, 325 F. Supp. 781 (M. D. Alabama 1971).

"The parent may be motivated to ask for such institutionalization for a variety of reasons other than the best interest of the child, himself, i.e. the interest of other children in the family, mental and physical frustration, economic stress, hostility toward the child stemming from the added pressures of caring for him, and perceived stigma of mental retardation. The retarded child's best interest may well lie in his family and in the community, but theirs may not lie in keeping him" (C. W. Murdock, "Civil Rights of the Mentally Retarded," *Notre Dame Lawyer* 48 [October 1972]: 133).

13. In our survey when asked to number in order "who you feel should carry the major responsibility" for a decision "to allow certain severely damaged babies to die by withholding treatment," the physicians placed "the child's parents or legal guardians" at the top of the list, "the attending physician second," followed closely by "a hospital committee," while "Court of Law" and "Clergy" followed far behind.

14. D. S. Roberts, Justice of Superior Court, *Maine Medical Center and Martin A Barron, Jr., M. D.* v. *Lorainne Marie Houle and Robert B. T. Houle:* February 14, 1974.

15. R. Muir, Jr., J. S. C. Superior Court of New Jersey: In the matter of Karen Quinlan. November 10, 1975.

16. J. A. Robertson, "Involuntary Euthanasia of Defective Newborns: A Legal Analysis," *Stanford Law Review* 27 (January 1975): 213-269.

17. M. C. Weinstein and W. B. Stason, "Foundations of Cost-Effectiveness Analysis for Health and Medical Practices," *N. Engl. J. Med.* 296 (1977): 716-721.

This fascinating article from the Center for Analysis of Health Practices, Harvard School of Public Health, develops a technique of cost-benefit analysis based on quantified quality of life concerns expressed as a measurement of "quality-adjusted life years (QALYs)." In a companion article, Stason and Weinstein illustrate how their analytic technique can be used ". . . both to determine how resources can be used most efficiently within programs to treat hypertension and to provide a yardstick for comparison with alternative health-related uses of these resources" (M. C. Weinstein and W. B. Stason, "Allocation of Resources to Manage Hypertension," *N. Engl. J. Med.* 296 [1977]: 732-739).

If these techniques show promise in helping society develop priorities in the allocation of resources for health programs, it seems likely that they will be used to scrutinize many aspects of newborn intensive care.

18. Our survey showed broad support for the following propositions:

Physicians need not attempt to maintain the life of every severely impaired newborn infant simply because they have the technology and skill to do so; parents and physicians (in that order) should carry the ultimate responsibility for deciding whether or not to withhold treatment from severely impaired newborns (under circumstances where the physician disagrees with a parent's nontreatment decision, a court order mandating treatment may be sought); such decisions should be made on the basis of the best medical predictions concerning longevity and quality of life; decisions to treat or not to treat defective newborns are best made on a case by case basis within broad guidelines; public discussion and involvement of physicians with lay groups with these issues are "appropriate and/or necessary."

III.
LEGAL QUESTIONS

Glanville Williams

The Legal Evaluation of Infanticide

What is our moral reaction to infanticide, as evidenced in our legal institutions? Do we regard it as an ordinary murder or as something more
venial? Have there been any movements of thought on the subject?

Social anthropologists distinguish between infanticide and murder.
Infanticide is the killing of a new-born child committed by the parents or
with their consent. The killing of another man's child is, according to
this definition, simple murder; it is the killing by or on behalf of the
parent that raises special problems.[1]

Many primitive peoples practised infanticide (along with contraception and abortion) as a means of population control. Infanticide is a
more crude and wasteful method of keeping down numbers than contraception. On the other hand, if we put aside ethical considerations for a
moment, infanticide has the advantage that it does not endanger the
mother, as unskilled abortion does, and as some primitive contraceptive
practices are capable of doing.

Non-Christian peoples are frequently found to resort to infanticide
not merely from sheer necessity but from considerations of convenience,
such as the woman's fear that her husband may be faithless while she is
nursing the child. Even such sophisticated folks as the Greeks and

A revised version of Chapter I of *The Sanctity of Life and the Criminal Law* (N.Y.: Alfred
A. Knopf, 1967).

Romans of classical times, as well as some of the Germanic tribes, practised infanticide for prudential reasons, where the uncontrolled growth of the family would have left the parents less able to provide for the established children. Among nearly all people who give the parent this *jus vitae necisque*, the decision has to be made at birth, and is in some cultures rendered easier by not counting the child as a full human being or a member of the tribe until some ceremony has been performed. Thus in Athens the child could be exposed before the Amphidromia, a family ceremony at which the child was carried by its nurse around the hearth and thus received religious consecration and its name.[2]

What seems appalling to the modern mind about the behaviour of the Athenian Greeks of the classical age, and of the Romans too, is perhaps not so much their custom of getting rid of newly born children for whom they could not provide, as the means they adopted for doing so. The practice of exposing the baby meant that death was the most merciful fate that might befall it: often the child might be picked up by someone, and reared for slavery or prostitution. This appalling callousness and want of parental feeling, as it seems to us, was not condemned by any writer; Plato and Aristotle positively approved of it, at least for weakly and deformed children. 'Habit,' wrote Sir J. R. Seeley, 'dulls the sense and puts the critical faculty to sleep. The fierceness and hardness of ancient manners is apparent to us, but the ancients themselves were not shocked by sights which were familiar to them. To us it is sickening to think of the gladiatorial show, of the massacres common in Roman warfare, of the infanticide practised by grave and respectable citizens, who did not merely condemn their children to death, but often in practice, as they well knew, to what was still worse—a life of prostitution and beggary. The Roman regarded a gladiatorial show as we regard a hunt; the news of the slaughter of two hundred thousand Helvetians by Caesar or half a million Jews by Titus excited in his mind a thrill of triumph; infanticide committed by a friend appeared to him a prudent measure of household economy.'

The change in moral outlook was very largely, if not entirely, the work of the church; it proceeded partly from an interpretation of the Sixth Commandment, and partly from the theological doctrine of the soul. The last needs a word of explanation. The mere supposition that the newly born child had a soul could not have given rise to a prohibition of infanticide, since, even if the child had a soul, and even if it were further supposed that souls after death were divinely punished for sin (either by pain or by annihilation), the soul of a child killed shortly after birth could evidently not be punished for any sin committed during life, because it had had no opportunity of sinning. From this point of view, infanticide might have been regarded as a positive benefit to the child, in excluding the possibility of damnation. Christian theology countered this argument in advance by adopting the theory of an original sin that could be removed only by baptism. Adam sinned by breaking God's command-ment, and this sin vitiated his seed and so was transmitted to his children and his children's children; Christ the Redeemer offered the opportunity of escape from the consequences of sin, both original and acquired; but the ceremony of baptism was the essential cure for original sin. If a child died after baptism he was capable of going to heaven; if before, the best that Catholic theology could do for him was to assign him to limbo, ex-cluding him from heaven.

There were, indeed, always some theologians who disputed this opinion, holding that a loving God would punish a person only for his own sin, and not for the sin of Adam; but their opinion was powerfully and effectually combated by Saint Augustine of Hippo.[3] According to Augustine, every man who is born, whether in wedlock or even in for-nication or adultery, is God's work; but he is born damned, born into the grasp of the devil, unless he is lucky enough to be baptized before death.

The enormous sin in slaying a newly born child, then, was not so much depriving it of life, as depriving it of the opportunity of baptism, whereby its soul passed without salvation, with all that implied for the life to come. It followed from this opinion that killing a newly born child was a worse sin than killing a baptized adult.[4]

Although Saint Augustine is still regarded with great veneration in the Roman Church, and his doctrine has never been explicitly disavowed, it is not always actively maintained. Saint Thomas Aquinas suggested the possibility of salvation for an infant who died before its birth,[5] and it is not a long step from this to admitting the possibility of salvation for the infant who dies unbaptized. There is a minority but gradually spreading opinion among Catholic theologians to lend support to this view, one suggestion being that the infant at the actual moment of death receives a 'supernatural illumination' which gives him the status of a morally adult person, enables him to understand the doctrine of original sin and the importance of baptism, and so leads him to wish for baptism, which wish has the same effect as baptism in water. The exponents of this 'liberal' doctrine avoid the imputation of heresy by emphasising that they do not claim theological certainty for their position, but merely suggest a possibility; consequently, their suggestion is not intended to undermine the doctrine of original sin or the importance traditionally attached to the practice of baptism in the Catholic church.[6]

Outside the Catholic community there has been a greater abandonment of the old ideas. The story of Adam has, since Darwin, come to be recognized as allegorical, and when the great majority of biologists are firm against the inheritance of acquired characteristics, the doctrine of original sin might seem to be deprived of its last vestige of rational support. It is true that neither the doctrine of original sin nor the practice of infant baptism has been totally abandoned by those churches that have been accustomed to profess them;[7] but most Protestants now look upon baptism as a traditional way of affirming a religious belief rather than as a necessary step for the receipt of divine grace. At the least it may be said that the ancient ideas are no longer regarded with the assurance that makes them an acceptable support for a rule of the criminal law. Criminal prohibitions cannot, at the present day, be founded upon supernaturalism of any kind. It is true, again, that the idea that the killing of any human being is in some way a sinful interference with the divine purpose persists, but the former religious view of infanticide seems now to be a strange inversion of values. Infanticide appears to our generation to be a crime less heinous than ordinary murder. Even if there is no social justification for the act, the killing of babies who are not old enough to experience fear is different from the murder of adults. This opinion was well and courageously expressed by Mercier, an English physician, in 1911.

> In comparison with other cases of murder, a minimum of harm is done by it . . . . The victim's mind is not sufficiently developed to enable it to suffer from the contemplation of approaching suffering or death. It is incapable of feeling fear or terror. Nor is its consciousness sufficiently developed to enable it to suffer pain in appreciable degree. Its loss leaves no gap in any family circle, deprives no children of their breadwinner or their mother, no human being of a friend, helper or companion. The crime diffuses no sense of insecurity. No one feels a whit less safe because the crime has been committed. It is a racial crime, purely and solely. Its ill effect is not on society as it is, but in striking at the provision of future citizens, to take the place of those who are growing old; and by whose loss in the course of nature, the community must dwindle and die out, unless it is replenished by the birth and upbringing of children.[8]

In this passage Mercier evidently puts aside religious eschatology and considers infanticide exclusively from a secular or utilitarian point of view. Even granting this assumption, however, not everyone will agree with his concluding remark that infanticide is in fact a racial crime, or, if it is a racial crime, that this is the only secular reason for its place in the law. Whether infanticide is racially an evil depends on the demographic situation at the time—in conditions of overpopulation infanticide is a positive benefit to existing society. But there is another reason for suppressing child-slaying within the utilitarian ethic, namely that the happiness of the child is to be considered. Worldly happiness, after all, is impossible without a life in which to enjoy it. It is worth observing that utilitarianism, though it originated as a secular system of ethics, is not devoid of a metaphysical foundation. As an ethical theory it depends upon an intuited premise, namely that the greatest happiness of the greatest number of human beings is the supreme good. This intuited premise or categorical imperative may be given any one of a number of interpretations, according to the opinion of the particular moralist who puts it forward. For example, the premise may assert that every child, once born, is entitled to its portion of happiness; or the premise may even accord moral rights to unborn children. On the other hand, it may take a restrictive view and make the moral question depend on the prospect of happiness enjoyed by the particular infant. According to the latter interpretation, severely handicapped infants may rightfully be put to death. General opinion is certainly far from taking this position at the present time, and all religions with any pretence to an ethical content are firmly against it. Even the modern infidel tends to give his full support to the belief that it is our duty to regard all human life as sacred, however disabled or worthless or even repellent the individual may be. This feeling, among those who do not subscribe to any religious faith, may sometimes be in fact a legacy of their religious heritage. Although morals need not logically depend on a transcendental faith, the system of morals professed in a society with a long religious tradition is likely to be coloured by that religion.

I am not clear in my own mind that this general opinion, whether religious or secular, on the subject of the sanctity of life justifies the punishment of a mother who, finding that she has given birth to a viable monster or an idiot child, kills it. I venture to doubt whether society has the right to stand in judgment upon a mother placed in this terrible predicament. We need to remember that toleration is a virtue, and that even a strictly moral person may be flexible in his morality, exercising his judgment upon the facts of the particular case and not looking exclusively to the rules of a legalistic ethic. Regarded in this spirit, an eugenic killing by a mother, exactly paralleled by the bitch that kills her misshapen puppies, cannot confidently be pronounced immoral. And where this certainty is lacking, should not liberty prevail?

However, even if this suggestion is not immediately put aside as impossibly wicked, there are difficulties in providing for the situation by law. Any acceptable scheme for the euthanasia of severely handicapped babies would involve the co-operation of the medical profession, which might not be forthcoming; in any case the proposal would occasion acute religious conflict. The most practicable course is, therefore, to recognize that the condition of the child killed by the parent may be the strongest mitigation of legal guilt. Courts have now obtained a very wide discretion to discharge without punishment where this appears to be expedient or where there are sufficiently weighty circumstances of mitigation.

'MONSTERS'

There is, indeed, some kind of legal argument that a 'monster' is not protected even under the existing law. This argument depends upon the very old legal writers, because the matter has not been considered in any modern work or in any court judgment. Bracton, writing under Henry III, seems to say that a monster is not a human being, '*quia partus monstruosus est cum non nascatur ut homo*'. Bracton is, understandably, not precise in his definition of a monster, and makes the utterly fanciful remark that a monster utters a roar, whereas a true child of Eva will cry the note E or A. He is careful to add, however, that a child is not accounted a monster merely because it has the wrong number of fingers or joints, or is crooked or hump-backed or has twisted limbs or otherwise has its members useless.[9] This passage is substantially repeated by Blackstone,[10] who says that a monster, who in any part evidently bears the resemblance of the brute creation, cannot be heir to any land, albeit it be brought forth in marriage; the reason, he says, is too obvious, and too shocking, to bear a minute discussion. Blackstone is here undoubtedly expressing the belief that a monster is the product of an animal paternity. Locke relates that women were known to have conceived by apes, 'if history lye not',[11] and it was an easy inference that monsters were the result of such an unnatural liaison. This error detracts from the legal authority that the passage in Blackstone might otherwise have possessed. Yet the question still remains whether it is not permissible both morally and legally so to define a human being as to exclude the grosser sports of nature. This is only another illustration of the fact that value-judgments have somewhat arbitrary limits, and are frequently hard to separate from questions of meaning. Since the determination of meaning must be made by men, the limits of the value-judgment must be settled by men, too.

Fortunately, the question whether a monster is human has small practical importance for the most extreme cases, because the acephalous, ectocardiac, etc., monster will usually die quickly after birth. This beneficent tendency of nature is assisted, in Britain at any rate, by the practice of doctors and nurses, who, when an infant is born seriously malformed, do not 'strive officiously to keep alive', even though they do nothing positive to kill it. The infant will be left unattended for a number of hours; a normal child will survive for quite a time without attention, but the monster usually dies. On rare occasions such a monster will live. It may belong to the fish stage of development, with vestigial gills, webbed arms and feet, and sightless eyes. The thing is presented to its mother, who struggles to nurture it for a few months, after which she sends it to a home. In one such case of which I was informed, a mother who already possessed a normal child gave birth to a viable monster. Both monster and normal child contracted influenza with a high temperature; the doctor treated the normal child but not the monster. The monster nevertheless survived.[12]

It seems probable that the medical practice is unduly cautious, and that a creature that is clearly a monster in the old-fashioned sense could lawfully be put to a merciful death. This appears to be a reasonable deduction from the rule stated by Bracton and the other institutional writers that a monster is not a man. It is true that they give or imply the wrong reason for it; but the same rule might be approved for a better reason. The only possible objection, apart from the extreme view that even a monster is the abode of an immortal spirit, is the difficulty of drawing the line; but all moral and legal rules require a line to be drawn somewhere. It may be noticed that even the Catholic religion, which is very strict on these matters, does not assert that a monster is certainly a man. According to the old Roman ritual, 'a monster which does not belong to the human species should not be baptized; if there is any doubt, it should be baptized with this condition expressed: "If thou art a man, I baptize thee, etc." '[13] The new Code of Canon Law, Canon 748, makes a slight change, providing that all monsters are to be baptized conditionally. Canon Henry de Dorlodot explained the Canon on the ground that it was a counsel of safety, the decision whether a monster is a human being frequently presenting difficulty. 'Canon 748 supposes that it is at least probable that some monsters born of woman are not really human: otherwise there could be no point in prescribing only conditional baptism.'[14]

As so often happens, the religious approach muffs the moral problem. Obviously the thalidomide babies, however terribly deformed, were human, as some of them have abundantly proved by courageously facing their handicap. The question a sensible person would ask is not verbal but moral: is the child so severely affected that one should make a judgment on its behalf that life will be too great a burden for it? On this, opinions will differ. The most important question is whether society is justified in punishing those who return an affirmative answer and kill the child.[15]

Siamese twins present a special case, though they are treated in medical works as a species of monster. Here the medical practice is to attempt a severance, notwithstanding the risks involved. Either the twins are successfully unlocked, or they die.[16]

Monsters are sometimes the unintentional result of medical treatment, as with the thalidomide disaster. Another scientific advance tends even more seriously in the same direction. The use of nuclear energy, by increasing radiation, is probably increasing the number of mutations, which are usually harmful. It may well be that in the future this also will add to the number of malformed and imbecile children brought to birth, and so give greater urgency to the legal and ethical problems involved. A serious increase in the number of degenerate children might well force mankind to a policy of 'weeding out' which is at variance with our present humanitarian outlook.

THE TREATMENT OF THE MOTHER

Let us assume that these problems are put aside, and that the act of infanticide is regarded not only as absolutely wrong but as subject in all instances to the control of the criminal law. There remains the question of treatment or punishment. On this matter the ecclesiastical doctrine had a calamitous result. For many centuries in the countries of Europe the mother who killed her child, perhaps when her mind was disturbed or when she was overcome by grief or worry at having given birth to a bastard, was, under the stimulus of the church, put to death. Some countries provided special pains for her: in Germany and Switzerland, the criminal code of Charles V provided the almost unimaginable punishment of burying the miserable offender alive with a pale thrust through her body.[17] The Christian church has often been praised for the heightened value that it attached to human life: the debit side of the account—the frightful punishments practised by our professedly Christian ancestors, in gross misinterpretation of the plain teachings of the New Testament—must not be overlooked. Bertrand Russell described moral progress as consisting in the main of widening the bounds of human sympathy. Our forefathers were so solicitous for the dead that they sometimes forgot all decency and humanity to the living.

Even today, in England and in a number of other Commonwealth countries that retain a fixed punishment for murder, if once the mother is convicted of murder, the court has no problem to consider, because she must be sentenced to life imprisonment as in any other case of murder. The law follows the religious view and refuses to regard the killing of an infant, even by the mother, as belonging to a lower legal category than the murder of an adult. However, the attitude proves to be impossible to maintain in practice. When a capital sentence was the rule in England for murder, there was no question after 1899 of its being carried out in these circumstances, so that it became nothing more than a devilish kind of jest, though the unhappy woman herself might not realize that the working of the law was kindlier than its professions. This fact, together with the frequent refusal of juries to convict mothers of the murder of their children, prompted in England a widespread desire for change in the law.

One line of approach is to treat the mother who kills her child at a time when she has not fully recovered from the effects of the birth as not fully responsible for her actions. To some extent the desired result can be achieved if she adduces evidence of insanity, but there are various difficulties with this. In the first place, the rejection in most Commonwealth jurisdictions of the defence of 'insane impulse' means that the insanity defence is a limited one. It is available where the mother kills her child in a confusional state, for then she may be taken as not knowing what she is doing, or that it is wrong; but a depressive psychosis, which is by far the most usual psychosis during and immediately after pregnancy, may have no legal effect upon responsibility. In the second place, the disturbance in the mother's mind which causes her to kill her child is not necessarily a psychosis (insanity). She may merely have been suffering from the obvious stress of having an illegitimate child; or there may possibly be an endocrine lack. In the third place, the insanity plea is disliked because of the supposed stigma of an insanity verdict, and the fear of committal to a state mental hospital of the security type. A way out of these difficulties was suggested in England by the Criminal Code Bill of 1878, which, as amended, proposed the institution of a new offence to meet the case.[18] The proposal did not reach the statute book till 1922.[19] The Infanticide Act of that year was replaced with amendments by an Act of 1938, which provides that where a woman by any wilful act or omission causes the death of her child being under twelve months, but the balance of her mind was disturbed by reason of her not having fully recovered from the effect of giving birth to the child or by reason of the effect of lactation consequent upon the birth, she shall be guilty of infanticide, punishable like manslaughter. This means that she can be sentenced to imprisonment for life—a purely theoretical possibility, too fantastic for consideration, when the woman has been found to have been deranged. In practice she is generally treated with great leniency, being discharged without punishment, or put on probation, or sent to a local hospital where she will be discharged as soon as the doctors think she has recovered.

It may be observed at this point that the use of the term 'infanticide' in the statute is unfortunate, because the statutory definition is narrower than the meaning adopted by anthropologists, who do not confine 'infanticide' to cases of mental unbalance. The offence designated in the English statute might better be called by some such distinguishing name as 'puerperal infanticide', but the specification of a whole year as the time during which the child may be deemed to be newly born shows a desire to interpret the puerperal period with the utmost generosity.

The Act, which has been adopted in some other parts of the Commonwealth,[20] has undoubtedly effected a great improvement in practice. On the other hand, from a technical point of view, it may be said to be an illogical compromise between the law of murder and humane feeling. It recognizes the inadequacy of the present law of insanity for the case of infanticide, and has the advantage of sparing the woman the agony of a murder trial when there are strong circumstances of mitigation. Yet it allows the conviction as for crime of a woman who may in fact have been afflicted by the puerperal mania, a real temporary insanity. If the woman was insane, the verdict should be one of insanity, and conviction should be out of the question. Under any rational system it should be better to be acquitted of an offence on the ground of insanity than convicted of another offence of slightly lesser degree.[21]

When the outcome of an infanticide trial is merely probation or discharge, this is perhaps not a serious criticism. But the Act does not save the woman, who may already be in great mental distress, the humiliation, disgrace, and agony of a formal trial before judge and jury. Although the charge in England first comes before examining magistrates, they have no power to deal with it summarily with the consent of the defendant, even though the facts are such that it is certain that she will receive a nominal sentence only. This is a legacy of the ancient and discredited doctrine that the criminal law must look to the abstract nature of the crime rather than to the circumstances in which it was committed and the treatment needed by the offender. Another criticism is that the Act leaves it optional to the prosecution to charge either murder or infanticide as it thinks fit. Generally, in circumstances covered by the Act, the charge will be infanticide. But sometimes the prosecution has frustrated the whole object of the Act by charging murder. An instance occurred in England during the last war, when a woman killed her newly born child and her own mother connived at the act. But for the participation of the older woman, the mother would probably have been charged with infanticide. As it was, the prosecutor imagined that he would be met with legal difficulty if he brought in an accessory to a charge of infanticide;[22] so he indicted both women for murder. The defendants were convicted, and, despite a strong recommendation to mercy by the jury, lay in the condemned cell for nine weeks before being reprieved.[23]

The Infanticide Act applies only for a year after the birth. It sometimes happens that a mother, loving her children, kills them to save them from the menace of insanity, disease, or desperate poverty, perhaps after trying in vain to have them taken off her hands by a children's home. Such a woman had, under English law as it stood before 1957, to be charged with murder, and, on conviction, sentenced to death, even though executive clemency was certain to intervene. But the law worked capriciously, because the outcome of the case depended on the leniency of the jury and the temper of the judge. In 1949 a charge of murder against a young married woman ended with a probation order. Her husband falling out of work, she had got into arrears with hire-purchase instalments; this preyed on her mind, and she was found unconscious with her child in a gas-filled room. The mother recovered, but the child did not. The mother was charged with murder of the child, pleaded guilty to manslaughter, and was placed on probation. This was a sensible solution, because it enabled the probation officer to help the unfortunate woman with her difficulties.[24] Contrast the outcome when, in 1953, a Scotswoman was charged with the murder of her child. In just over seven years of married life she had had six children. Her own upbringing was bad, both parents being heavy drinkers. The birth of the fifth child, Thomas, was very difficult and the mother was thenceforward liable to violent fits of temper. Thomas was delicate and sickly, often crying and moaning, and one day his mother, finding that he had woken up the baby, beat him to death with a broken chair-leg. Thomas was then a little over two years old. The mother's record as to the other children, in care and treatment, was good beyond the average. She was convicted of manslaughter and received the terrible sentence of six years' imprisonment.[25]

Some of the foregoing criticisms of the Act presuppose that the woman is in fact mentally disordered, as the Act assumes. But an opposite, and paradoxical, criticism is that the mental disorder is often a myth. Dr. D. J. West, who studied cases where married women had killed their children, found no particular association with the period following childbirth.[26] As for the reference to the state of lactation, there is no evidence that this is associated with mental disturbance. The association is a legal fiction, designed to extend the lesser offence to the full year after childbirth.[27] In reality, the operative factors in child-killing are now seen to be generally the stress of having to care for the infant, who may be unwanted or difficult, and personality problems; these affect the father as well as the mother, and are not confined to a year after the birth.

The Infanticide Act has reinforced feelings of sympathy for a woman who uses violence against her child, but only within its terms. If she kills the child, everyone assumes, on slight evidence, that she was mentally unbalanced by reason of the birth or lactation; does not the Act say so? But if the woman botches the killing and merely injures the child the Act does not apply; she will be charged with attempted murder or wounding with intent, and is quite likely to go to prison. Or if a mother kills both her newborn baby and an older child the Act does not save her from a charge of murder in respect of the older child, notwithstanding that any mental disturbance from which she suffered affected both killings. By English law she can now set up a defence of "diminished responsibility" in these cases. This was a Scottish invention introduced into English law by the Homicide Act 1957, and since adopted in other parts of the Commonwealth. It enables mental unbalance to reduce a charge of murder to one of manslaughter, and thus gives an opportunity for the wise and merciful treatment of any parent charged with the murder of a child of any age. But again the reduction of responsibility follows in law from the mental disturbance, not merely from mitigating factors connected with the relation of parent and child.

No legislation like the Infanticide Act is found in the United States, but the problem is somewhat alleviated by the possibility of finding second-degree murder. This does not entirely dispose of the problem, because there are frequently minimum periods of imprisonment of some severity, which can, however, be evaded by the use of probation. The experts in criminal law at Columbia University informed me that no full studies have been made of the way in which infanticide is actually treated by the American courts, and much depends upon the degree of enlightenment of the judge and jury. In an Alabama case of 1948, a mother who was convicted of murdering her newly born child received a sentence of twenty years' imprisonment; happily, the conviction was reversed on appeal for lack of evidence, but there was no animadversion upon the terrible sentence that the trial court had thought fit to impose.[28] Severe sentences naturally lead to a refusal on the part of juries to convict, and this has in turn led law enforcement officers to consider the desirability of something like the English infanticide legislation.[29]

In conclusion, a plea may be made for a greater exercise of the discretion of prosecuting authorities to refrain from prosecuting. The law makes a number of simplified moral judgments and enforces them on the ground of the public interest in social conduct. To a large extent these rules of conduct can be fitted to the individual case by adjustment of the punishment or treatment, or discharge without punishment. But one element in the legal process is ineluctable—the distress of mind caused to the offender by being summoned before a court, particularly where this involves much publicity in the Press. This reinforces the argument that a legal inquisition into conduct is not justified on moral or religious grounds if no sufficient social purpose is to be served.

Notes

1. See *Encyclopedia of the Social Sciences*, s.v. 'Infanticide'.
2. *Enc. Soc. Sci.*, s.v. 'Infanticide'; Westermarck: *The Origin and Development of the Moral Ideas* (London, 1906), I, 393ff.; Lecky: *History of European Morals*, 3rd. ed. (London, 1911), 24ff.; W. W. Tarn: *Hellenistic Civilization*, 3rd. ed. (London, 1950), pp. 92, 100; Cameron in 46 *Classical Review* 105 (1932); William L. Westermann: *The Slave Systems of Greek and Roman Antiquity* (Philadelphia, 1955), p. 86.
3. Augustine's principal writings on the subject were his *On the Baptism of Infants* and *On the Grace of Christ and on Original Sin*. Among the texts that he quoted were Rom. v, 12 ('Wherefore, as by one man sin entered the world, and death by sin; and so death passed upon all men, for that all have sinned'); John iii, 5 ('Except a man be born of water and of the Spirit, he cannot enter into the kingdom of God'). Augustine was, of course, well aware of other texts which he might have used to support the opposite conclusion, e.g., the passages in Jeremiah and Ezekiel asserting that if the fathers have eaten sour grapes, the children's teeth will not be set on edge.
4. Lecky: *History of European Morals*, 3rd. ed. (London, 1911), pp. 23-4; Westermarck: op. cit., 411-12.
5. Lecky: *History of the Rise and Influence of the Spirit of Rationalism in Europe* (London, 1904), I, 360, n. 2.
6. For a full discussion and bibliography upon the 'liberal' view, see Fr. Peter Gumpel, S. J., 'Unbaptized Infants: May They Be Saved?' (1954) 72 *The Downside Review* 341, (1955) 73 *ibid.* 317.
7. A survival of the older ideas may be seen in the English Book of Common Prayer, which forbids the burial service to all who die unbaptized—even though infants—as well as to those who die excommunicate or have laid violent hands upon themselves. In the American Book of Common Prayer the first prohibition applies only to unbaptized adults.
8. Mercier: *Crime and Insanity* (London, 1911), pp. 212-13; cf. his *Crime and Criminals* (London, 1918), pp. 193-4. Much the same argument had earlier been propounded by Bentham (*Theory of Legislation*, p. 264).

For an argument that the approach to child-killing should be social, e.g., by assisting the unmarried mother, see J. W. Jeudwine: *Observations on English Criminal Law* (London, 1920), Chap. 10.
9. Bract. f. 438a-b; cf. ibid., ff. 5a, 70a; he is not, however, speaking of homicide, which he does not consider in this connection. See also Coke upon Littleton, f. 7b.
10. Blackstone: *Commentaries*, II, 246.
11. Locke: *Essay Concerning the Human Understanding*, III, Chap. 6, s. 23.
12. Many examples of monsters from medical and general literature are given by Theodrick R. Beck and J. B. Beck: *Elements of Medical Jurisprudence*, 11th ed. (Philadelphia, 1860), pp. 422ff.
13. Quoted by William Reany: *The Creation of the Human Soul* (New York, 1932), p. 196. For a Protestant opinion that a monster is not human see E. L. Mascall: *Christian Theology and Natural Science* (London, 1956), p. 283.
14. See his discussion in E. C. Messenger (ed.), *Theology and Evolution* (London, 1949), 278-80.
15. For the criminal proceedings in Belgium which attracted much attention and resulted in an acquittal by the jury see Philippe Toussaint, *Le Procès de Liège* (Brussels, 1963).
16. For example, in February 1955 an operation was performed in London to separate twins joined at the crown of their heads but perfectly healthy. Both children died after the operation.
17. Westermarck: op. cit., p. 412.
18. See the *Report of the Criminal Code Commission of 1879*, p. 251. See also *Report of the Royal Commission on Capital Punishment, Cmd. 8932 of 1953*, pp. 57-9.
19. It had been anticipated in Natal by Act No. 10 of 1910, s. 9, which created a special offence of infanticide where the child was killed within a week of the birth.
20. See *Report of the Royal Commission on Capital Punishment, Cmd 8932 of 1953*, p. 447.

21. The offence of infanticide presents, indeed, one particular legal difficulty. Sometimes when a woman is charged with infanticide the facts may show that she is exempted from responsibility under the McNaghten rules, as when she acts in a state of automatism. For an instance, see William C. Sullivan: *Crime and Insanity* (London, 1924), pp. 96-7. In such cases it seems that the verdict should be one of insanity. Such a verdict is one that all parties to the case wish to avoid, and it was perhaps the intention of Parliament to enable it to be avoided.

22. There was in fact nothing to prevent the mother of the child being convicted of infanticide, and her own mother being convicted of murder, acting through a semi-innocent agent.

23. 6 *Howard Journal* 184 (1944-5). An Australian judge ruled, on legislation similar to the English, that the Crown should not indict for murder where a woman kills her newly born infant and the facts reveal an absence of premeditation, but should confine the charge to infanticide: Barry J. in Rex v. Hutty [1953] V.L.R. 338.

24. 113 *Justice of the Peace Journal* 337.

25. A brief account of the case (*Regina* v. *Hampton*) appeared in *The Times* (London), July 22, 1953.

26. *Murder followed by Suicide* (London, 1965), 147.

27. Glossary of Mental Disorders and their Classification (World Health Organization, 1974) 27 confines 'psychosis associated with childbirth' to 'unspecified psychoses that have occurred within 6 weeks following delivery.'

28. Singleton v. State, 33 Ala. App. 536, 35 S. 2d 375.

29. The *Annual Report* of the Attorney-General for Massachusetts for the year ending January 17, 1894, p. 12, contains the following passage: 'One of the capital cases tried during the year illustrates anew the difficulty of securing the conviction of a woman charged with the murder of her infant child. Under the existing law the Grand Jury and the prosecuting officer, though having the power to indict for manslaughter, are logically and morally bound to indict and try such cases, if appearing to be malicious, as for murder, which leads upon conviction to the penalty of death or imprisonment for life. This is liable to result in a failure of justice which might be avoided if the penalty were less severe. Some of these cases are of great hardship and appeal strongly to the sympathies of the jury, as, for example, when the mother has been seduced and abandoned by the father of the child; and in many of them, even in the absence of extenuating circumstances, the evidence is not of such a character as to procure a conviction of murder, though there may be no substantial doubt of the guilt of the accused. There is also high medical authority for the belief that some of these homicides are due to the mental disturbance which sometimes accompanies childbirth, rendering the mother more or less irresponsible for her conduct. For these and other reasons, both of justice and humanity, I suggest the expediency of providing that such homicide, even if appearing to be done with legal malice, may in the discretion of the Grand Jury and the prosecuting officer, be indicted as manslaughter instead of murder.' I am indebted to Professor Joseph Goldstein, who is working on the treatment of the criminal insane, for bringing this Report to my notice and allowing me to use it.

Leonard J. Weber

In Defense of the Legal Prohibition of Infanticide

It is to be expected that a serious re-examination of infanticide legislation has begun. We have grown increasingly aware of the fact that medical intervention sometimes extends life without healing or curing; much, much importance has been placed on the question of whether or not death may not be more desirable than continued life for some individuals. There is a growing conviction, it seems, that the law should permit or even authorize death in some cases because of the condition of the patient. Concern for what the law requires by way of treatment has been focused on one important area, the intensive care nursery.

In addition, recent court rulings on abortion seem to raise questions about legal rights and responsibilities in regard to infant care. Abortion rulings stress the right of mothers to freely decide the fate of the unborn without state intervention. Legislation regarding child care stresses the responsibility of the state to intervene to protect the child, even from his or her parents. It is natural to wonder whether or not the emphasis on parental privacy may not have implications for child care legislation.

In the current reappraisal of child care legislation, I would like to argue a case for the legal prohibition of infanticide. I am convinced that the most benefit will accrue to society by the enforcement of clear laws against the killing of human infants, regardless of their physical or mental condition.

Before making the argument, however, it is necessary to explain what is meant by "infanticide." It seems to be one of those terms, like "euthanasia," that is open to different interpretations and, therefore, should probably never be used without explanation. For some, infanticide is involved in any situation in which the maximum effort to prolong a child's life is not made. For some, infanticide implies a cold, calculated decision to murder an unwanted child. For others, the term is properly used to describe all cases of direct killing of infants and some cases of withholding treatment that could extend a child's life.

The term is used here in the third sense. Infanticide means the killing of infants, and killing means causing death or depriving of life. Some cases of withholding treatment are the moral (and, hopefully, legal) equivalent of killing; some are not. I would like to see the term infanticide used to describe, and the law used to prohibit, those actions and those omissions that can be considered killing without unduly stretching the meaning of the word. It is sometimes argued that we should stop "perpetuating the fiction that withholding treatment is ethically different from terminating life."[1] To some extent, it is a fiction: there is no significant moral difference between giving a baby a lethal injection and withholding permission for surgical correction of duodenal atresia, with the result that the baby starves to death (as in the famous Johns Hopkins case). On the other hand, it is also something of a fiction to say that every case of death when life could have been prolonged is killing, and is caused by human action or neglect. There are times when the most appropriate response is to care for a child as he or she dies, rather than desperately trying to prolong a life to the exclusion of really human caring. In those situations, that kind of a response should not be considered killing or infanticide.

It is not the purpose of this essay to provide guidelines for distinguishing between those cases where withholding treatment should be considered killing and those where it should not.[2] It is only important here that it be clear that support for laws against infanticide does not mean a desire that we be legally impelled to prolong life in all cases.

The discussion that follows presumes an intensive care nursery context. I am talking about mercy infanticide rather than infanticide involving healthy children. Laws against mercy infanticide are necessary, I am convinced, if we are going to preserve our social health and welfare as a people. That does not mean, however, that actions of this sort cannot be distinguished legally from infanticide without mercy. To recognize legally, for example, that there is a significant difference between mercy killing and killing for personal gain would probably make mercy killing laws less harsh and more enforceable.

The law should clearly prohibit infanticide; it should prohibit killing by direct intervention or by the withholding of appropriate curative treatment. To permit parents or others to decide to bring about death for their children because of their condition will have serious detrimental consequences for society.

INFANTICIDE AND SOCIETY

We ordinarily think of laws as regulators of behavior. And that they are. But we need to recall that one of the ways in which laws have an impact upon the quality of life in a society is through their educative role. They are a factor in shaping the values and attitudes of many citizens, and those values and attitudes are more responsible for restricting undesirable behavior than the legal punishments attached to that behavior.

The relationship between values, on the one hand, and criminal law, on the other, is not a simple one. Certain values need to be present in the first place before laws are enacted. But the social expression of approval or disapproval that is a law itself acts as a very important factor in the development of attitudes in society. Most Americans living in the middle of the nineteenth century, long accustomed to the legal enslavement of one race of men by another, were not inclined to see the institution of slavery as immoral or unacceptable. Most Americans living today, long accustomed to living in a society in which slavery is treated as a most serious crime, clearly find slavery totally unacceptable. Our values have changed profoundly over the years in this regard, and the law has had a significant role in changing those values.

What would happen if we would legally permit infanticide? What would be the likely, long-range impact upon our social values? How would such laws affect our respect for life? Laws are desirable or undesirable in terms of their consequences, and the impact that laws have upon such values as respect for life is a most important social consequence.

In view of the probable long-range consequence to society of permitting mercy infanticide, I think a very strong case can be made for prohibiting it. Since infants are not capable of making a rational choice of death for themselves, infanticide cannot be considered a voluntary decision on the part of the child. Given that consideration, and given as well the basic "right to life" proposition accepted in our society, the legal acceptance of infanticide would have to be accompanied by the propagation of one or both of the following social doctrines: (1) that some children are so abnormal that they should in reality be considered nonpersons; (2) that those who have severe physical or mental handicaps do not have the same right to life as those who are healthy. Both doctrines have profound implications for the wellbeing of society.

The Supreme Court's ruling on abortion (*Roe* v. *Wade*, 1973) partially, at least, resolved the problem of abortion in terms of who is a human person. It held that a human fetus is not a person, in the Constitutional meaning of the term, during the first two trimesters. Given that precedent, there is some likelihood that attempts to change laws in order to permit infanticide will include the argument that some infants, because of their handicaps, do not have the capacities (for example, for self-awareness and rationality) necessary for them to be considered human beings.[3] If some infants are not persons, it is not a violation of a human life or a human good to bring about their deaths.

If this is the doctrine that would be taught by the legal acceptance of infant mercy killing, it would, I fear, have some very serious and undesirable consequences. Workers for social justice have long argued that the only way that we can hope to achieve justice is to recognize that everyone is equal, regardless of race or religion or nationality or condition. To totally exclude some (because of reasons of health) from those human beings who have rights and enjoy the protection of laws is to abide by a policy of discrimination that may have important implications for other relationships in society. Discrimination and the deprivation of fundamental human rights because of differences have long been part of human history. (It is easy to think of examples such as racial slavery and the persecution of the Jews.) Before we begin to declare some others less than human, we should make sure that we are aware of the role of such labeling in human experience.

If the capacity for rationality, for example, is to be considered a criterion of humanness, will there not be a tendency to think of those who exhibit only minimal rationality as less human than others? Any sort of criteria which excludes some members of the biological species from human rights would almost inevitably result in discrimination among the rest on the basis of who is "more human" and "less human." Those discriminatory attitudes would, in turn, be reflected in our social practices.[4]

The other social doctrine that might be taught by the removal of the legal prohibition of mercy infanticide is that the lives of some human beings do not deserve the same protection as the lives of others. If we permit the killing of severely handicapped infants without defining them as nonpersons, then the law would be saying that the right to life and the prohibition against killing depend upon the condition of the one being killed. It is obvious that this, too, involves a tremendous potential for encouraging injustice. We would be establishing a policy that encourages and supports unequal treatment of unequals.

The argument is sometimes made that we have to put the focus on the "quality of life" rather than on the simple fact that one is an alive human being. There are, of course, advantages to the quality of life approach; it reminds us that it is not enough that we do not kill, that we must be concerned as well with what kinds of lives persons live. But to kill some because the quality of their lives is not what we consider minimally acceptable involves in itself a policy that would be harmful to the quality of life of many in our society. I suspect that Karen Lebacqz is quite correct in her judgment regarding the selective abortion of deformed fetuses: "In the long run, this violation of fundamental rights of equal treatment is a more serious threat to the 'quality of life' of all of us than the birth of numerous children with defects will ever be."[5] And this threat becomes increasingly more serious when we move beyond selective abortion to selective infanticide.

If the laws of the states permit killing because of some deformity or handicap, society is encouraging all of us, through those laws, to harden our hearts in regards to deformities. As we begin to bring death to those who have handicaps of a type that we may earlier have been able to tolerate, we (in the words of R. A. Burt) "are pushing along in barely perceptible steps the internal psychological processes which permit us one day rationally, coolly, bloodlessly, to consider what today seems wildly beyond possibility."[6]

If we withhold legal protection from infants who are severely handicapped, we will be punishing by death those who, through no fault of their own, are victims. There has always been a tendency in societies to use the technique of blaming the victim, to justify unequal treatment by finding defects in the victims of inequality (women are not capable of rationality, black culture is inferior, etc.). Removing the legal prohibition against infanticide would give social support and encouragement to the practice of justifying *our* actions in terms of the defects of the victims. I do not think that we can do that without doing great damage to the cause of justice and equality.

It has been said (and I think with accuracy) that the moral strength of a people can be measured by the way they treat the weak and defenseless. We sometimes look at history and take pride in thinking that society has, over the centuries, developed a more sensitive and responsible attitude toward the unfortunate. Mercy infanticide constitutes a reversal of that development.

FREEDOM OF CONSCIENCE

In a discussion of the possible legal solution to almost any problem, the question of freedom of conscience must be raised. Would a restrictive law be one that imposes the moral position of some on those who have a different moral opinion, with the result that some can only follow their own sincere consciences at the risk of serious legal penalities? Especially in questions such as mercy infanticide, where one's position on the value of the life of the handicapped infant may be closely related to his or her ethical and religious values, it is important that consideration be given to the question of freedom of conscience.

Sometimes the argument for freedom from state intervention in cases of infant care implies that the infant is not a human person and, therefore, the decision is truly a private one for the parent, a decision involving no one else. This essay has already considered the designation of handicapped infants as nonpersons and argued that that is a dangerous social policy.

At other times the argument for freedom from law is based upon a particular understanding of the proper function of law in a morally pluralistic society. According to this legal philosophy, it is best for the law to be as permissive as possible when there is serious disagreement about the moral acceptability of a particular type of behavior. Let me conclude this essay with a response to this position.

It is evident to me that there are many who are convinced that infanticide is, in some circumstances, the most responsible and moral way of dealing with the situation of handicapped infants. The question is truly one on which there is a difference of moral opinion. Furthermore, I agree that we should, provided the price is not too high, devise laws that permit persons to act according to their own best consciences. Nevertheless, I cannot conclude that infanticide should be permitted by law. This is one case in which the price to society for total freedom of conscience is just too high.

The law is a tool to be used to try to achieve the most desirable, or the least undesirable, consequences for society. What we consider a good law depends on what we think are desirable consequences and what we perceive to be the actual consequences of the law. It is often necessary to give up one desirable consequence in order that another, more important one, be protected. That is the situation here. The loss to society in terms of lives destroyed, the reduction of respect for life, and the encouragement of discriminatory practices is ultimately of greater significance than the loss of some freedom to follow one's conscience. When not given some necessary legal limitations, freedom becomes permission for the strong to impose their wills on the weak.

It is a sound principle of law that parents do not have a right to do whatever they want with their own children. We as a society have the obligation to protect children from the abuse of parents, regardless of what good intentions those parents may have. There is no doubt that supporters of mercy infanticide are well intentioned, but the law cannot focus as much on intentions as it does on consequences.

Notes

1. John M. Freeman, "Is There A Right to Die—Quickly," in *Moral Problems in Medicine*, ed. Samuel Gorovitz et al. (Englewood Cliffs, N.J.: Prentice-Hall, 1976), p. 356.

2. I have found the traditional ordinary/extraordinary means distinction helpful in determining when withholding means is the equivalent of killing. See Leonard J. Weber, *Who Shall Live? The Dilemma of Severely Handicapped Children and Its Meaning for Other Moral Questions* (New York: Paulist-Newman, 1976).

3. Much attention has been aroused by Joseph Fletcher's "Indicators of Humanhood: A Tentative Profile of Man," *The Hastings Center Report* 2 (November 1972).

4. Weber, *Who Shall Live?* p. 77.

5. Karen Lebacqz, "Prenatal Diagnosis and Selective Abortion," *The Linacre Quarterly* 40 (May 1973): 126.

6. Robert A. Burt, "Authorizing Death for Anomalous Newborns," in *Genetics and the Law*, ed. Aubrey Milunsky and George J. Annas (New York: Plenum Publications, 1976), p. 440.

Arval A. Morris

Law, Morality, and Euthanasia for the Severely Defective Child

Advances in the health sciences and in medical technology can be a mixed blessing. They can be used to help us lead vital, full, and robust lives. That is the view of modern medicine that most of us prefer. But, there is another one. The recent advances also can be used to prolong a mere biological existence—one without vitality, health, or any opportunity to know or enjoy the minimum satisfactions or pleasures basic to ordinary human life. For example, with today's "team" approach in medicine, using modern mechanical monitoring capabilities, intravenous hyperalimentation, ventilatory support systems and elemental diets, staged surgical technics, and other new methods, modern medicine can "salvage" many infants who would have died shortly after their birth twenty-five, or even five, years ago. Modern medicine can also sustain the "life" of dying persons (it really only prolongs their acts of dying), by propping up the young or old "subjects" on pillows or encompassing them within cocoons of oxygen. The young survive as long as they can marginally tolerate an oral or intravenous diet of amino acids and sugar and a number of tubes inserted into them. For many, the most probable prospect is either death or another operation, and nothing more. The MA-1 respirator provides a common example of a machine readily available in most American hospitals. The respirator provides air to a person's lungs on a controlled volume basis and also has a "sigh volume" capacity, which is a periodic increase in the volume of air that purges the lungs of any excretions or accumulations of fluids. The MA-1 respirator automatically takes over the breathing function whenever an infant or an adult does not breathe spontaneously. It can save the life of a person. But, it also can maintain the respiratory function indefinitely, even when there is little, if any, chance that the respirated "person" will recover his ability for spontaneous respiration. What prospect do persons in this latter type of situation have of ever enjoying the minimal satisfactions of basic, ordinary life?

The threshhold level of the basic opportunities needed to enjoy a minimum amount of human goods necessary to constitute life in the sense of "ordinary human life" is difficult to define with perfection, but they have been significantly if not completely described by Philippa Foot:

> The idea we need seems to be that of life which is ordinary human life in the following respect—that it contains a minimum of basic human goods. What is ordinary in human life—even in very hard lives—is that a man is not driven to work far beyond his capacity; that he has the support of a family or community; that he can more or less satisfy his hunger; that he has hopes for the future; that he can lie down to rest at night. Such things were denied to the men in the [Soviet] Vyatlag camps described by Dmitri Panin; not even rest at night was allowed them when they were tormented by bedbugs, by noise and stench, and by routines such as body-searches and bath-parades—arranged for the nighttime so that work norms would not be reduced. Disease too can so take over a man's life that the normal human goods disappear. When a patient is so overwhelmed by pain or nausea that he cannot eat with pleasure, if he can eat at all, and is out of the reach of even the most loving voice, he no longer has ordinary human life in the sense in which the words are used here. And we may now pick up a thread from an earlier part of the discussion by remarking that crippling depression can destroy the enjoyment of ordinary goods as effectively as external circumstances can remove them.[1]

Because of recent advances in science and their applications to modern medicine, techniques can be used to prolong life merely as a biological existence without any reasonable possibility for "ordinary human life." This is a relatively recent phenomenon. Because of it we have reached a new condition in human life that calls for a new consciousness. We now must reevaluate one of the Western world's most basic premises, and we must recognize that mere life, itself, is not always a good. Where it is not, the hope for a speedy end naturally arises in the consciences of people of compassion and justice. In such circumstances, the question of euthanasia, properly understood, becomes a pressing legal and moral question, and it is forced upon us by our current stage of development in medical technology. But euthanasia is an emotional subject and is poorly understood.[2] It has many dimensions. There are at least voluntary, involuntary, and nonvoluntary euthanasia, with each of the three categories perhaps admitting a further distinction between passive and active euthanasia.[3]

VOLUNTARY EUTHANASIA

Voluntary euthanasia appears to be best understood and to have the widest degree of public acceptance in American society. The passive type of voluntary euthanasia is typified as the "right to die." It merely requires that in certain situations no heroic medical measures shall be taken in order to sustain life. Whatever life-sustaining mechanisms that may be in use are switched off, just as they were in the case of Karen Ann Quinlan. Passive voluntary euthanasia seems to have greater public approval than the active type, which requires a positive act designed to terminate biological existence. But active voluntary euthanasia merely amounts to legally assisted suicide, and when euthanasia, itself, is properly understood, active voluntary euthanasia is also widely accepted. The principle of voluntary euthanasia encompasses the active and passive varieties, but it applies only to the right of an *adult* person (1) who is incurable; (2) who is not within the reach of any cure or medical treatment that may reasonably be expected to come into effective existence during his life expectancy; (3) who is expected to suffer severe physical and/or psychological pain; (4) who is in full command of his faculties; and (5) who declares (or previously has made a written declaration) that in such circumstances he either declines all further medical treatment (passive euthanasia) or desires to have his life ended by a physician, pursuant to his own intelligent request, under specific conditions prescribed by law, and by painless means (active euthanasia). Because acts of voluntary euthanasia, both passive and active, can be acts of mercy carried out for the sake of the subject, and because the subject, being in a normal mental condition, not only voluntarily requests euthanasia but also needs it in order to avoid pain and suffering, it is generally agreed that acts of voluntary euthanasia can be morally justified on grounds of individual freedom, charity, and justice. However, the voluntary principle, itself, is limited, applying only to adults who are in rational command of their faculties. Thus, on principle, voluntary euthanasia is not available for nonrational or mentally disturbed adults who are unable to give rational, informed consent, nor can it properly be applied to any severely defective child, regardless of the objective need or the subjective desire for it.[4]

INVOLUNTARY EUTHANASIA

Lying at the other extreme, far away from morally justified voluntary euthanasia, is involuntary euthanasia, which can be either active or passive. By active involuntary euthanasia I mean a situation where a person who molests no one and is in command of his faculties demands by word or simply by his everyday deeds that he be let alone to live, but nevertheless, he is intentionally killed without there being any justifying reason. Normally and properly, we condemn such killings as murder. The reason is that rights and duties exist between all human beings, and one of the most important rights that an ordinary human being can have is the right to life itself. In the ordinary situation, the right to life imposes a duty of noninterference on others that is owed to each person by every other person. Thus, it is obvious that if a person who respects the rights of others and is in rational command of his faculties declares or otherwise manifests his desire that he does not wish to die, that he does not wish to be interfered with, then no one can justifiably administer active involuntary euthanasia to him. To do so is to commit murder; it violates his fundamental right to life itself, and is morally unjust. However, although active involuntary euthanasia is clearly and properly condemned and ruled out as unjust, the same condemnation may not be equally applicable to passive involuntary euthanasia. The justness of the latter depends upon whether the subject of passive involuntary euthanasia has a relationship involving special rights and duties with others that goes beyond the duty of noninterference.

Clearly, the subject of passive involuntary euthanasia is equally owed the duty of noninterference by others. But, in this context, the complete observance of the duty of noninterference, and nothing more, may really mean that the duty's recipient knowingly will be left alone to starve to death involuntarily, a practice that can be identified as passive involuntary euthanasia. This practice arguably may   justified or unjustified, depending upon additional circumstances regarding rights and duties. For example, adults morally owe a duty of care and maintena e to their elderly parents who, in turn, have corresponding rights of support against their adult children. In such circumstances, it would be morally unjustified, as well as uncharitable, for an adult child to refuse to share his food with his starving elderly parents knowing that they desired and needed food, thereby practicing passive involuntary euthanasia on them. On the other hand, while it may demonstrate a reprehensible lack of charity, it would not necessarily be an act of moral injustice for a total stranger, who may be rich or poor, knowingly to refuse to share his family's food with the starving elderly couple. During the recent famines in sub-Sahara Africa many peoples and nations refused to share their food supplies with the needy peoples of other nations, who subsequently starved to death, and they believed their refusals to have been justified, but surely they could not believe themselves to have been kind or charitable.[5] Thus, the justice or injustice of passive involuntary euthanasia depends upon the character of the relationship of rights and duties that exists between the subject and other persons.

NONVOLUNTARY EUTHANASIA

Both voluntary and involuntary euthanasia, whether of the active or passive varieties, crucially depend upon a special characteristic: that of a person being in command of his faculties, thereby possessing the rational ability to declare or to manifest a desire on whether he wants to die or not. Voluntary euthanasia requires consent to death and involuntary euthanasia requires manifested, but minimally ordinary, resistance to death, so that it is known to be against the subject's competent will. Neither voluntary nor involuntary euthanasia can have any direct application to severely defective newborn infants. They cannot be said to be capable either of giving or refusing their voluntary consent. That is the major reason why the law requires that a parent or legal guardian give informed consent before his child undergoes an operation. Severely defective newborn babies present an especially difficult problem for euthanasia. The issues here are materially different from those involving euthanasia for adults who capably can manifest their intentions one way or the other. The situation of severely defective children is neither voluntary nor involuntary, but is aptly described as one involving the question of nonvoluntary euthanasia. Is it ever justified to practice nonvoluntary euthanasia, whether passive or active, on severely defective newborn infants or young children? The answer turns on the specific nature of the problems, and on a proper understanding of the meaning of "euthanasia."

THE SPECIFIC NATURE OF SOME PROBLEMS OF SEVERELY DEFECTIVE CHILDREN AND SOME MEDICAL PRACTICES

It is a fact today that in most of the world's developed countries medical care for newborn infants has become increasingly effective and complex. As scientific knowledge and medical technology have advanced, obstetricians and pediatricians can now intervene successfully to maintain the lives of high-risk or defective newborn babies who previously would not have survived. Nature no longer blindly takes her toll. The immediate and active application of medical technology can result in newborn survival where death would previously have resulted. Equally, but conversely, by withholding medical treatment an infant's death can result that, perhaps, could have been prevented.

The life or death of high-risk, defective newborns rests, in the first instance, on the decision of the attending physician. Generally, however, the practice in a hospital delivery room, and elsewhere, is to provide immediate emergency care to severely defective newborns in deference to the widely held but popularly unexamined beliefs that life, whatever its nature, is a good and that the duty of all medical personnel is to preserve human life, whatever its form. When these beliefs are conjoined with emergency life-sustaining mechanisms that immediately are available in modern hospitals, the lives of many severely defective newborns automatically are maintained when, surely, they would have died had their delivery been at home, as was the custom fifty years ago, when life-sustaining machines were not immediately available. But, in modern hospitals where the medical treatment of the severely malformed neonate is successful, or even where none is offered, life may endure, but that life may not be ordinary life. It may be biological only, being severely handicapped and drastically truncated in its potential for human development, satisfaction, and happiness. Severely defective newborns who have survived may have little or no capacity to love or to be loved, and many of them will spend their lives in institutions that have been labeled as not much more than "dying bins." Severely deformed infants may never have the possibility of "ordinary human life," in the sense set forth above by Philippa Foot. Thus, because of modern medical technology and the widespread belief that all life is a good, within seventy-two hours after delivery the question frequently arises whether the life-sustaining medical machines should be switched off.

The failure or refusal to provide medical or other care to the defective newborn has occurred throughout the ages. Infanticide by exposure has roots that are lost in the mists of antiquity. But it is only recently that the practice of deliberately withholding medical treatment has been openly admitted and defended by modern physicians. In the *New England Journal of Medicine* in 1973, Doctors Raymond M. Duff and A. G. M. Campbell publicly broke the taboo, when they reported on forty-three severe cases of congenitally defective newborn infants in which heroic medical care was withheld and death ensued.[6] In this group of forty-three infants were fifteen with multiple anomalies, including various kinds of brain damage, eight with trisomy, eight with cardiopulmonary disease, seven with meningomyelocele, three with differing but severe central-nervous-system disorders, and two with short-bowel syndrome. In each case anguished parents in consultation with physicians, in what must have been a traumatic decision, concluded that the prognosis for any kind of treatment and rehabilitation that would lead to a meaningful life was either hopeless or extremely poor at best, and, therefore, further medical treatment would be discontinued. Since Duff and Campbell's initial report other cases have been made public, including a hearing that was held by the Senate's Subcommittee on Health, during which eminent physicians sought to justify the medical nontreatment of severely defective infants as good medical practice.[7] Thus, it is clear that nontreatment of severely defective newborns is becoming a widespread hospital practice in the United States and England, raising the questions whether the practice of nonvoluntary euthanasia, passive or active, is, in some sense, morally justified, and whether it ought to be explicitly authorized and regulated under a rule of law. To answer these questions adequately it is necessary first to have a clear idea of the meaning of

THE PROPER MEANING OF EUTHANASIA

Properly understood, euthanasia is a matter of deciding in favor of death on the ground that death is in the better interests and is preferable to life for the one who is to die. The crucial requirement is that the welfare of the recipient of euthanasia is the guiding criterion. Euthanasia is administered solely and exclusively for his sake, and for no one else's. This is the proper view of the matter. It merely expresses the new condition of human consciousness by recognizing that life itself is not always a good, irrespective of its nature. Popular speech recognizes as much when people say of a person that "he would be better off dead." This proper view of euthanasia—that it is solely for the sake of the subject—serves to distinguish it sharply from the murder that was disguised under the label of "euthanasia" and practiced in Nazi Germany by Hitler's doctors. A proper view of euthanasia is consistent with our ideals of respect for an individual's dignity and liberty and with an individual's claims to justice and charity.[8] This view of the matter rules out administering nonvoluntary euthanasia to severely defective infants (1) because they are not "persons"; (2) because they would cause greater suffering to others (parents, other family members and siblings, nurses or doctors) than the benefits that they, themselves, would derive from continued living; or (3) because they would be an economic or social burden. On this humane and proper view of euthanasia the question whether it can be administered to any severely defective newborn turns exclusively on whether one can reasonably say that it is being administered for his own sake; that is, "would he be better off dead?"

THE MORALITY OF NONVOLUNTARY EUTHANASIA APPLIED TO SEVERELY DEFECTIVE CHILDREN

Recognizing that life itself is not always a good, and that, indeed, in some situations it can be an evil, then under what circumstances can it confidently be said that some severely defective newborns should die while others should be subjected to heroic medical measures in order that they might have the opportunity to live? No fully satisfactory and infallible general standard applicable to all cases can be offered. Each child's case must be judged on its own merit. The above quotation from Philippa Foot is a good beginning statement of the criteria for judgment.[9] But, except for categories such as anencephalic babies (those with no, or only a partial, brain and no top to the skull), the case of each severely deformed newborn or defective child should be evaluated on his own merits in light of his particular disease or condition, its severity, its known course of development, its capacity to produce pain and suffering, and the child's individual prognosis.

The known courses of development of some diseases can give fairly clear pictures of biological existences that are so lacking in opportunities to enjoy a minimum amount of human goods that they cannot be said to permit human life in its basic and minimally ordinary sense. Examples of such biological existences whose only possibility is painful suffering, in addition to anencephalic newborns, are children afflicted with Lesch-Nyhan disease, which is characterized by compulsive self-mutilation and severe mental retardation, and children afflicted with Tay-Sachs disease, which is characterized by progressively severe increases in spasticity, dementia, pain, and deprivation, and generally leads to death by the age of four or five; often such children are susceptible to aspiration pneumonia, which serves to intensify all the existing painful injuries of their short and marginal existences. Another example involves an infant whose gastrointestinal tract has been surgically removed after suffering volvulus and infarction, and who has had a central venous catheter inserted. Is it morally right to insert this "lifeline" which can support the "life" of this infant for a maximum period of, perhaps, two years, so long as the infant remains tethered to an infusion pump? I think there will be widespread agreement that the use of the modern arsenal of modern technology in an attempt to prolong the biological existences of defective newborns such as the ones just described is a misguided or wrongful act that results in cruelty, is contrary to the better interests of the infant, and violates the important maxim of medical ethics, *primum non nocere*, that, first and foremost, one should do no harm. The truth is that in such circumstances death is a good and the prolongation of life is an evil.

On the other hand, the question becomes more difficult when considering other debilitating deformities whose known course of development is not as clearly destructive as the diseases described above. They may or may not permit a child to enjoy a basic and minimally ordinary life. But even in the case of the more difficult predictions, procedures can be employed that may produce results that will bring the more difficult cases within the ambit of systematic knowledge so that reliably tested decisional rules-of-thumb can be created. Spina bifida, a birth defect of uncertain origin, serves as an example. The spinous process, a portion of the vertebrae, is split in children with spina bifida and part of the spinal cord is malformed and may be extruded either into a blisterlike bag or outside it, if the bag has ruptured; hydrocephalus is common. Most frequently, such children are paralyzed and suffer from bladder and bowel infections, malfunction, or incontinence. It is not unusual for them to be mentally retarded. In the past, most spina bifida children died from meningitis after a short life because of the spinal cord's continual exposure to infection. Today, however, medical technology can sustain the life of many children who previously would have died. Modern techniques include straightening the spine, closing the lesion, draining the hydrocephalus if one has developed, and eliminating infection through medical treatment. The result is that a large percentage of the children having spina bifida survive, but a large number of them are physically handicapped and mentally retarded.

Dr. John Lorber of Sheffield, England, has specialized in a clinic devoted to the care of children who have spina bifida. After twelve years of following a policy based on the premise that all life is always a good, thereby trying to sustain the life of every newborn having spina bifida, he reviewed the records of his spina bifida clinic and concluded that its policy was in error. He proposed that a new policy of selective medical treatment should be instituted. Basically, Lorber recommended a set of rules created in light of the massive therapeutic experiment that had taken place in Sheffield. It turns out that even though a good specialist cannot identify, with certainty, the future maximum amount of disability, he is able to identify the minimum degree of future handicap that will ensue from spina bifida by analyzing the degree to which the newborn is paralyzed, his head circumference (identifying the probability of hydrocephalus), the degree of spinal curvature, if any, other major birth injuries, and any other associated gross or congenital anomaly.[10] Dr. Lorber believes that his rules should govern the selective medical treatment of spina bifida cases because they have been designed to work in the better interests of the children, by making medical treatment available to those children who have some opportunity to develop the capacities needed to enjoy the minimal amount of human goods that can be said to constitute a basic level of ordinary human life. His rules for decision are well tested, and if followed, they clearly are superior in accuracy to the more or less ill-informed decisions currently being made by parents in consultations with nonspecialist, local physicians.

Dr. Lorber's selective treatment rules have the further advantage of not automatically applying medical technology to every case of spina bifida, thereby unnecessarily extending the biological existence of some children who will surely die anyway, and in the process subjecting them to the morbidity of multiple surgical and other pain-producing medical measures. Surely euthanasia, in some instances passive and in others active, in the cases of children identified for nontreatment under Lorber's rules and in the cases of children who are born anencephalic or who are afflicted with Lesch-Nyhan or Tay-Sachs disease would prove a boon to them, just as it would for young children who develop cancer—metastic cancer, involving the lungs, the liver, the brain, and other vital organs that slowly and painfully cease to function when afflicted with cancer. An application of euthanasia in these cases would invoke the proper meaning of the term because reason indicates that euthanasia would be for their sakes and for no one else's. Of these children we can truly say that "they would be better off dead." Moreover, since one can appropriately hold, on grounds of justice, that no duty of treatment is owed to these children because to treat them would be to do them harm by engaging in a useless, pain-producing act, and since one can also hold on grounds of charity that it is better that the pain and suffering of the severely defective children be terminated as quickly and as mercifully as possible, it would appear, therefore, that these cases, and other cases like them, are properly cases of nonvoluntary euthanasia of severely defective children and that it is morally justified. Indeed, it may be morally compelled.

THE LEGALITY OF NONVOLUNTARY EUTHANASIA FOR SEVERELY DEFECTIVE CHILDREN

Although nonvoluntary euthanasia of severely defective children is morally justified and may even be required as an act of mercy, and although, as reported by Drs. Duff, Campbell, and others, its practice is becoming widespread in hospitals in the United States and Great Britain, nevertheless, the practice currently may be illegal. One thorough study in 1975 analyzed the practice in relation to possible criminal liability under our existing laws:

> Although the courts have not yet ruled directly on the criminal liability of persons who refuse ordinary life saving medical care for defective infants [they have ruled parents criminally responsible for killing defective offspring, see U.S. v. Repouille, 165 F.2d 152 (2d. Cir., 1947)] under traditional principles of criminal law the omission of such care by parents, physicians, and nurses creates criminal liability. The crimes committed may include murder, involuntary manslaughter, conspiracy, child abuse or neglect.[11]

One must be cognizant, too, that there always are several witnesses in a delivery room and elsewhere in a hospital. This fact is graphically illustrated by the case of *Commonwealth* v. *Edelin*,[12] decided by the Supreme Judicial Court of Massachusetts. Dr. Edelin performed an abortion by hysterectomy on a seventeen-year-old, unmarried woman whose gestational period was variously estimated as ranging from seventeen to twenty-six weeks. He made no attempt to apply the arsenal of modern medical technology to the fetus in order to save its "life." For his conduct, Dr. Edelin was indicted for manslaughter of the fetus and convicted after trial during which his fellow health professionals were obliged to testify. On appeal, all six Justices who heard the case agreed that there were errors committed during the trial, and five of the Justices further agreed that, as a matter of criminal law, Dr. Edelin should never have been judged by the jury because, in his specific case, there was insufficient evidence showing that he in any way had acted in a "wanton" or "reckless" way. But, given the initial success in this case at the trial and given the general principles of criminal liability, it is likely that Duff and Campbell, and other physicians whose practice is to consult with parents on whether to withhold medical treatment, probably neglect to consider or to advise the parents of their, and of the physicians, potential criminal liability when they collectively decide (conspire?) to withhold medical treatment.

As the *Edelin* case illustrates, one should not conclude that no criminal prosecutions will ever be brought after such parent-physician consultation and after the proper administration of euthanasia to severely defective infants. The lack of prosecutions to date is probably explained by the fact of its low visibility: (1) prosecutors do not read medical journals, and most of them are unaware of the recent development of the practice; (2) neither doctors, nurses, other health professionals, nor parents complain to prosecutors about the practice; (3) the few prosecutors who do know of the practice, by exercising their discretion, currently refuse to prosecute probably (a) because of the nature of the anguish and the nature of the human problems involved, or (b) because a prosecution might be politically unpopular, or (c) because of the nature of the legal case and a lack of manpower, since some complicated and novel points of law are involved. Nevertheless, physicians, parents, and other health professionals should not conclude that they have nothing to fear from the law when they collectively decide to administer euthanasia to a severely defective child. As time passes and as the practice obtains a higher degree of visibility, it will surely be debated publicly. The right-to-life groups may well shift their attention from abortion to euthanasia, particularly if abortion receives greater public approval. All of these events appear highly probable; thus, it is likely that somewhere some few prosecutors will believe that they must bring some criminal prosecutions. Criminal cases will probably occur in the future, at least until the legal issues are clarified and resolved. That is why it is wise to anticipate this likely development and to make the needed changes in the law now.

THE LAW'S DEFECTIVE PREMISE

The laws that could culminate in criminal liability for the proper administration of euthanasia to a severely defective child share one common and basic premise with much of early medical practice in America and with dogmatically held popular beliefs against all euthanasia. This premise antedates and is made obsolete by the rise of modern health sciences and medical technology. The defective premise is that life, whatever its form, nature, or content, is necessarily and always a good, and that death, or any event that hastens death, is always and necessarily an evil and should be illegal. Law has a felt obligation to protect life to the fullest for each individual and seeks to assure each person's right to live out his life until its natural and inevitable end, which is legally defined as "cessation," meaning a total stoppage of the circulation of the blood and a cessation of all the animal and vital functions resting on blood circulation, such as pulse, respiration, etc. The problem is that, as commendatory as the law is in this regard, the law's basic premise applies only to the usual and ordinary person and was created with him in mind. As discussed above, this commonly shared premise is false. There simply is no plain, straightforward, and necessary connection between all human life itself, in each and every instance, whatever its character, and its always being a good. Ordinarily life is a good, and the usual person can enjoy at least a minimally ordinary human life and should receive the law's protection. But, life is not always a good in each and every instance. It is this class of extraordinary cases, few in number in the total population, in which life is not always a good. They are the proper concern of euthanasia. Thus, the primary change that is needed in the law, and elsewhere, is a modification of the commonly held basic premise that life, whatever its form, nature, or content, is always a good and that any act or event that hastens death is an evil and necessarily is a legal wrong.

THE BEGINNING WINDS OF LEGAL CHANGE

In the *Karen Ann Quinlan* case,[13] decided unanimously on March 31, 1976, the Supreme Court of New Jersey became the first court in the United States partially to modify the law's defective premise and explicitly to recognize that life, whatever its form, nature, or content, is not necessarily to be considered as always being a good and not always to be prolonged as long as possible. In doing so, the court boldly and correctly asserted that "the law, equity and justice must not themselves quail and be helpless in the face of modern technological marvels presenting questions hitherto unthought of," and that the distribution of responsibility between medicine and law "should however neither impede this Court in deciding matters . . . nor preclude a re-examination by the Court as to underlying human values and rights." It continued saying that court "determinations as to these [human values and rights] must, in the ultimate, be responsive not only to the concepts of medicine but also to the common moral judgment of the community at large." Then, in the course of its opinion, the court explicitly approved passive voluntary euthanasia and passive nonvoluntary euthanasia in certain circumstances, but only for adults.

Karen Ann Quinlan was an adult of twenty-two, not a severely defective child, when New Jersey's Supreme Court decided the case. For reasons that are unclear, she ceased breathing for at least two fifteen-minute periods on the night of April 15, 1975. She was given mouth-to-mouth resuscitation, rushed to a hospital, put in an intensive care section, placed on the MA-1 respirator, and there she stayed because all "attempts to 'wean' her from the respirator were unsuccessful and have been abandoned." The medical consensus was that Karen Ann Quinlan, in addition to being comatose, was also in a chronic and persistent "vegetative" state, having no awareness of anything or anyone around her; she existed at a primitive reflex level and could not survive at all without the assistance of the respirator. (This last medical belief proved to be false.) Despite this state of affairs it was the medical consensus, and the court found that under "any legal standard recognized by the State of New Jersey and also under standard medical practice, Karen Ann Quinlan is presently alive."

Confronted by the drastic condition of his daughter and her poor prognosis, and after making an anguished decision, Karen's father, Joseph Quinlan, a devout Roman Catholic, who had consulted with his priest,[14] petitioned the court (1) that he be appointed as guardian of Karen's property and person, and (2) that the guardianship, if permitted, should contain an express power authorizing him to order the discontinuance of all extraordinary medical procedures that were sustaining her vital processes and, hence, her life. Mr. Quinlan also asked the court to declare that if he were appointed Karen's guardian and if he ordered the discontinuance of all life-sustaining measures, then the local prosecutor should be barred from prosecuting him for any crime. The State Attorney General intervened and asked the court to deny Mr. Quinlan's petition and completely to reaffirm the state's interest in the law's mistaken premise that life, whatever its form, nature, or content, is necessarily a good and is always to be fully protected and prolonged. Finally, one of Karen's physicians asked for clarification of his legal and professional responsibilities if he were to remove Karen's life-sustaining measures because (1) Karen Quinlan was alive, and (2) the physicians in charge of the case had previously declined to withdraw the respirator because the prevailing medical practice, and hence, the professional duty of the physician, was that of not removing the respirator in cases like hers.[15]

Without discussing the matter directly, New Jersey's Supreme Court rested pat on its conclusion that Mr. Quinlan should be appointed Karen's guardian, on a proper view of euthanasia. It considered the case as one in which the litigation has to do, in final analysis, with her life, and the question to be decided was whether the court could authorize Karen's guardian to decide in favor of her death solely on the ground that death would be in her better interests and would be preferable to prolonging her life. Without revealing its criteria used in judgment, which I suspect was that the prognosis was so extremely poor that Karen Ann Quinlan would never again reach the threshhold level of basic opportunities necessary to enjoy a minimum amount of human goods necessary to constitute life in the sense of "ordinary human life," the court stated that it had "no doubt, in these unhappy circumstances, that if Karen were herself miraculously lucid for an interval (not altering the existing prognosis of the condition to which she would soon return) and perceptive of her irreversible condition, she could effectively decide upon discontinuance of the life-support apparatus, even if it meant the prospect of natural death." The court distinguished Karen's case from one of its previously decided cases in which it had ordered a blood transfusion in order to save a woman's life. The court pointed out that "most importantly," in the transfusion case, the patient was "salvable to a long life and vibrant health—a situation not at all like [Karen's] case." Indicating that it might disapprove of suicide and active voluntary euthanasia, the court explicitly recognized the legal right to passive voluntary euthanasia by any adult who is in command of his abilities and who is painfully and terminally ill:

> We have no hesitancy in deciding . . . that no external compelling interest of the State could compel Karen to endure the unendurable, only to vegetate a few measurable months with no realistic possibility of returning to any semblance of cognitive or sapient life. We perceive no thread of logic distinguishing between such a choice on Karen's part and a similar choice which, under the evidence in this case, could be made by a competent patient terminally ill, riddled by cancer and suffering great pain.[16]

This right to passive voluntary euthanasia, the court held, was grounded in the constitution's right to privacy which "is broad enough to encompass a patient's decision to decline medical treatment under certain circumstances, in much the same way as it is broad enough to encompass a woman's decision to terminate pregnancy under certain conditions." Thus, the court ruled against the law's mistaken premise and against the Attorney General's argument that the state has a legal and compelling interest in prolonging all life, whatever its nature. New Jersey's Court stated "that the State's interest . . . weakens and the individual's right to privacy grows [in importance] as the degree of bodily invasion increases and the prognosis dims," and that "ultimately there comes a point at which the individual's rights overcome the State interest"; thus, "it is for that reason that we believe Karen's choice, if she were competent to make it, would be vindicated by the law."

But, of course, Karen Ann Quinlan was incompetent to make any choices. "Nevertheless," the court concluded, "Karen's right of privacy may be asserted on her behalf by her guardian under the peculiar circumstances here present." This conclusion was necessary, the court believed, because "the only practical way to prevent destruction of [Karen's] right is to permit the guardian and family of Karen to render their best judgment; subject to the qualifications hereinafter stated, *as to whether she would exercise it in these circumstances.*"[17]

The *Quinlan* court next considered the physician's dilemma. On the basic point of medical responsibility the court concluded that:

> Physicians distinguish between curing the ill and comforting and easing the dying; that they refuse to treat the curable as if they were dying or ought to die, and that they have sometimes refused to treat the hopeless and dying as if they were curable . . . *many of them have refused to inflict an undesired prolongation of the process of dying on a patient in irreversible condition when it is clear that such "therapy" offers neither human nor humane benefit.* We think these attitudes represent a balanced implementation of a profoundly realistic perspective on the meaning of life and death and that they respect the whole Judeo-Christian tradition of regard for human life. No less would they seem consistent with the moral matrix of medicine, "to heal," very much in the sense of the endless mission of the law, "to do justice."[18]

The court then ruled that if Karen's guardian ordered that all life support measures be discontinued and, if the physician's view were that this order contradicted his professional obligations, or if this kind of problem should again arise in the future in some other but similar case, then, in that situation, a physician should share his professional responsibility. The court stated that a Professional Medical Ethics Committee should be created for each hospital, and it should consider all future cases and advise the physician on his professional obligations.[19] The *Quinlan* court underscored that this committee should be composed of diverse persons —physicians, lawyers, social workers, other health professionals, theologians, and others—and that "the most appealing factor" of this approach was "the diffusion of professional responsibility for decision, comparable in a way to the value of multi-judge courts in finally resolving on appeal difficult questions of law." The court believed that "such a system would be protective to the hospital as well as the doctor in screening out, so to speak, a case which might be contaminated by less than worthy motivations of family or physician." Moreover, it clearly ruled that "we would have no doubt that such decisions, thus determined to be in accordance with medical practice and prevailing standards, would be accepted by society and by the courts, at least in cases comparable to that of Karen Quinlan."

Finally, the court declared "that there would be no criminal homicide in the circumstances of this case . . . [because] first, . . . the ensuing death would not be homicide but rather expiration from existing natural causes, [and] secondly even if it were to be regarded as homicide, it would not be unlawful." Although it used some language to the contrary, New Jersey's Supreme Court avoided the active voluntary or nonvoluntary euthanasia questions by declaring that "there is a real and in this case determinative distinction between the unlawful taking of a life of another and the ending of artificial life support systems as a matter of self-determination." In the latter situation "a death resulting from such an act would not come within the scope of the homicide statutes proscribing only the unlawful killing of another."

Thus, New Jersey's Supreme Court expressly approved (1) passive voluntary euthanasia for a terminally ill, but rational adult, and (2) passive nonvoluntary euthanasia for Karen Ann Quinlan and for all other "cases comparable to that of Karen Quinlan," in which a guardian is appointed and voluntarily decides that euthanasia is genuinely for his ward's sake.

THE QUINLAN CASE AND SEVERELY DEFECTIVE CHILDREN

The Quinlan case is *not* a direct precedent, even in New Jersey, authorizing nonvoluntary euthanasia of severely defective children. The case does not preclude New Jersey's Supreme Court from taking such a step in the future, and it may well do so. While it is true that parents of severely defective children are in a legal position similar to that of Mr. Quinlan's guardianship of his adult daughter, it is also true that children do not have all the same constitutional rights as adults. No court has yet ruled that a newborn, or a child of thirty-six hours, or one of two years of age has a constitutional right to privacy. Thus, it is possible that in the case of a severely defective child the *Quinlan* case's constitutional foundation is lacking, and that parents, although equally guardians of their severely defective children, would be unable to exercise a nonexisting right to privacy on behalf of their child.

On the other hand, the case opens some new avenues. Once a physician has discharged his duty fully to "inform" (really to educate) an adult who is mentally competent, that adult generally has the option of accepting or rejecting the proposed medical treatment, and, indeed, as the *Quinlan* court ruled, that adult, if terminally ill, (or that adult's guardian) may refuse any and all treatment. But, if a child and not an adult is involved, then a parent can give his informed consent for medical treatment of his child, but if he rejects either the specifically recommended or any and all treatment, then that parent's decision rejecting treatment can be subjected to court review when either physicians or governmental authorities disagree with it. Thus, it can be seen that the *Quinlan* case lays the foundation for a new legal procedure that would permit a parent to give his informed consent for euthanasia if euthanasia is considered by physicians to be the most appropriate medical treatment and if it is believed by the parent to be in the better interests of a severely defective child, so long as there has been review of that parent and physician decision by a competent agency, say by a court or by a Professional Medical Ethics Committee.

The *Quinlan* case required the creation of a Professional Medical Ethics Committee. This requirement provides a vehicle for the generation of norms of professional responsibility for physicians in cases of severely defective children, responding to current problems created by modern medical technology in cases such as anencephalic newborns, or cases of children afflicted with Lesch-Nyhan or Tay-Sachs diseases or with cancer that has metasticized and affects the lungs or the liver or the brain or other vital organs that slowly and painfully cease to function. But, the inadequacy of the *Quinlan* case's approach, strictly construed, is that it ultimately leaves the final decision where it does not belong—in the hands of the physician—when it should rest in the hands of those parents who have been shown to love their children and to act for their welfare. Clearly, parents must participate in any decision about any aspect of medical treatment of their severely defective children, and they must be fully informed about the consequences of giving or withholding

155

consent. But, informed consent in the case of nonvoluntary euthanasia of a severely defective child is a matter that goes well beyond the usual informed consent, which merely involves the presentation of the possible complications of proposed surgery, length of hospitalization, the probable total cost, recuperative time, and other medical matters. In the case of nonvoluntary euthanasia, the parents must also talk with friends, religious or moral counselors, and others. Moreover, the value of a child's life is at stake and that means that neither the parents nor a Professional Medical Ethics Committee should have the sole responsibility for the decision. The responsibility should be spread among them and it should also include the child's attending physicians as well.

The *Quinlan* case points in the right direction. But, given the *Quinlan* court's aversion to active nonvoluntary euthanasia, even if it authorized passive nonvoluntary euthanasia at some future time, and allowed a decision to withdraw medical support mechanisms from severely defective newborns or children, that decision would be terribly cruel because it would merely leave the children to die either by starvation or by painful natural death processes as the child's disease takes its toll.

The *Quinlan* case is, therefore, neither a direct nor an adequate solution to the problems presented by severely defective newborns or by older children. It is an important straw in the wind. Its great merit lies in its partial reconsideration and in its partial reconstruction of the law's false premise that all life, whatever its form, nature, or content, is always a good and always is to be protected by the law and prolonged. Additionally, the *Quinlan* case, although not controlling, can be a useful foundation for an equivalent, a future test case that would involve a severely defective newborn or an older child. But, few parents will consider going through the agony and the legal procedures of a test case as did Mr. Quinlan, and fewer still will actually do it. Moreover, although in some social circumstances courts may be the only reasonable means available, their decisions necessarily are piecemeal and do not systematically attack the overall problem. Proper authorizing legislation, if it can be obtained, is much more thorough, complete, and desirable.

Notes

1. Philippa Foot, "Euthanasia," *Philosophy and Public Affairs* 6, no. 2 (Winter 1977): 85–112.
2. For discussion see, Glanville Williams, *The Sanctity of Life and the Criminal Law* (New York: Knopf, 1957), and Marvin Kohl, *Beneficent Euthanasia* (Buffalo, N.Y.: Prometheus Books, 1975).

3. The distinction between passive and active euthanasia (between withholding treatment and allowing a patient to die, and taking direct action to kill a patient) is not as clear as one might believe, nor is it true that passive euthanasia is always preferable, in every case, over active euthanasia. For discussion see, J. Rachels, "Active and Passive Euthanasia," *New England Journal of Medicine* 292, no. 2 (January 9, 1975): 78-80.

It seems clear to me that an "act" is required in both active and passive euthanasia. The difference is that the "act" in active euthanasia necessarily is done with the desire and intent to kill, but while switching off a respirator in passive euthanasia is also an "act," it may not necessarily be done with the intent to kill; yet, the expectation of the actor surely is that the most probable consequence of his act of turning off the switch will be death; thus, the difference between active and passive euthanasia is slight, lying in the distinction between an act while intending death, in the case of active euthanasia, and an act in which the actor may not intend death, but he surely is reasonably expecting it, in the case of passive euthanasia. This line of analysis appears to have been overlooked by G. Fletcher, "Prolonging Life," 42 *Wash. L. Rev.* 999 (1967), and G. Fletcher, "Legal Aspects of the Decision Not To Prolong Life," *J. of Am. Med. Assoc.* 203, no. 1 (January 1, 1968): 119-122.

4. For further discussion see, A. Morris, "Voluntary Euthanasia," *Washington Law Review* 45, no. 2 (1970): 239-271.

5. One writer states that although some people are urging "upon the world community the moral principle that all basic human needs ought to be recognized as *claims* . . . right now," it is nevertheless true that "in many cases, they cannot yet plausibly be treated as *valid* claims, that is, as grounds on any other people's duties" (J. Feinberg, "Human Rights," in *Moral Problems in Medicine*, ed. S. Gorovitz [Englewood Cliffs, N.J.: Prentice-Hall, 1976], p. 465).

6. Duff and Campbell, "Moral and Ethical Dilemmas in the Special Care Nursery," 17 *New Engl. J. Med.* 289 (1973): 890.

7. United States Senate Committee on Labor and Public Welfare, Subcommittee on Health, *Hearings*, 93rd Cong., 2nd. Session, June 11, 1975.

8. For further discussion see, P. Foot, "Euthanasia," pp. 85-112.

9. Also see J. Fletcher, "Indicators of Humanhood: A Tentative Profile of Man," *The Hastings Center Report* 2, no. 5, Hastings-on-Hudson, New York, Institute of Society, Ethics and the Life Sciences, November 1972, pp. 1-4, and J. Fletcher, "Ethical Aspects of Genetic Controls: Designed Genetic Changes in Man," *New England Journal of Medicine* 285 (1971): 776-783.

10. J. Lorber, "Results of Treatment of Myelomeningocele," *Developmental Medicine and Child Neurology* 13 (1971): 290-300; also see J. Lorber, "Early Results of Selective Treatment of Spina Bifida Cystica," *British Medical Journal* (October 27, 1973): 204, and J. Lorber, "Selective Treatment of Myelomeningocele: To Treat or Not To Treat," *Pediatrics* 53 (March 1974): 307.

Dr. Lorber's criteria have been strongly challenged by researchers who would substitute a different set of criteria, see, e.g., D. Shurtleff, et al., "Myelodysplasia: Decision for Death or Disability," *New Engl. Jour. Med.* 291 (1974): 1005, and D. Shurtleff, "Meningomyelocele: The Price of Treatment," *Yearbook of Pediatrics*, (1973): 332-336, but compare, M. Tooley, "Abortion and Infanticide," *Philosophy and Public Affairs* 2, no. 1 (1972): 37. No part of this article turns on taking sides in the debate or proposing new criteria. It is sufficient for my purpose that commonly agreed-upon criteria exist and where there is dispute over a criterion, then to insist on action that "errs," if that word is correct, on the traditional side of sustaining life.

11. J. Robertson, "Involuntary Euthanasia of Defective Newborns: A Legal Analysis," *Stanford Law Review* 27, no. 2 (1975): 213-269, at p. 217. For example, in the treatment of his patients a physician is required to exercise the degree of care, knowledge, and technical skill that is ordinarily possessed and exercised in the same or similar situations by the average member of the medical profession practicing in his field. If the physician is a specialist, then he must use skills superior to those of a general practitioner and demonstrate his use of that special degree of skill normally possessed by the average specialist in his par-

ticular field, whether he be specialized in a particular disease, injury involved, or in attending to a special organ, having regard for the present state of relevant scientific knowledge. These considerations define the content of a physician's duty that establishes his particular legal obligation to his patients. The medical obligation is related to the standards and practices prevailing in the profession generally or in its specialized branches.

12. 359 N.E. 2d 4 (1976).

13. 70 N. J. 10, 355 A2d. 647 (1976).

14. Bishop Casey's position validated that of Mr. Joseph Quinlan. After reviewing the doctrines of the Roman Catholic Church and a specific pronouncement on the general area by Pope Pius XII on November 24, 1957, Bishop Casey concluded that "the decision of . . . [Mr.] Quinlan to request the discontinuance of this treatment is, according to the teachings of the Catholic Church, a morally correct decision."

15. See note 11 for the source of the physician's concern.

16. In re: Karen Ann Quinlan, 355 At12d 647, 663 (1976).

17. Emphasis supplied.

18. Emphasis supplied because of its relevance to severely defective children. The court also stated that it "would have to think that the use of the same respirator or life support could be considered 'ordinary' in the context of the possibly curable but 'extraordinary' in the context of the forced sustaining by cardio-respiratory processes of an irreversibly doomed patient."

19. The court took this idea from Karen Teel's article, "The Physician's Dilemma: A Doctor's View: What the Law Should Be," *Baylor Law Review* 27, no. 6 (1975): 8-9.

IV.
SUFFERING AND THE VALUE OF LIFE

John Donnelly

Suffering: A Christian View

Jean De La Fontaine remarked in the seventeenth century (Fables, I, 16) that it is "better to suffer than to die: that is mankind's motto." In the late twentieth century it would appear many philosophers are prepared to reverse this shibboleth to read "better to die than to suffer." For a good number of contemporary philosophers the prevention of suffering has achieved higher priority as a value claim than the preservation of life.

I wish to unravel in this paper, by focusing on Soren Kierkegaard's gospel of suffering, the contention that seems to underlie discussions on the morality of infanticide, namely, that intense, prolonged, and often incurable suffering, either by the infant directly or guardian indirectly (or both), is bad and there is no redeeming value in such suffering. My aim is to see if this contention is true. I believe I can show that the contention is at least arguably false.

Writing about a hydrocephalic child, possessed of a huge head, lying in bed wildly swinging his arms to beat himself (even wearing padded gloves), O. Ruth Russell writes:

> Is it not perfectly clear that such a defective child should be painlessly put out of his misery either at birth, or as soon thereafter as diagnosis makes it possible for physicians to predict with reasonable certainty that life can be nothing but tragic?[1]

163

A view similar to Russell's is held by H. Tristram Engelhardt who, in speaking about the "injury of continued existence," postulates a duty to prevent (prolonged) suffering. The presupposition behind such views seems to be that nonexistence is preferable to a negative "compromised" existence.[2] Engelhardt writes:

> In the case of a child with meningomyelocele, one might argue that when the cost of cure would likely be very high and the probable lifestyle open to attainment very truncated, there is not a positive duty to make a large investment of money and suffering. One should note that the cost here must include not only financial costs but also the anxiety and suffering that prolonged and uncertain treatment of the child would cause the parents.[3]

Pace Russell, Engelhardt, et al., the proposition "suffering is evil" is not necessarily true. We have the evidence of St. Paul, Franz Brentano, and Mother Teresa for this point, as well as the more silent testimony of many others. Indeed, it may not even be contingently true in all instances. For example, the infant suffering from some currently incurable physiological ailment (e.g., cystic fibrosis, sickle cell anemia, etc.),[4] and his guardians, could be thankful for his/her affliction, which enables them to develop traits of character and mental sets not so readily fostered in a healthy body or nontragic situation.

Marvin Kohl, who has often insightfully outlined the dangers of the slippery slope argument, seems to somewhat unwittingly slip into it by claiming that "indifference to suffering tends to beget indifference or cruelty."[5] Kohl's remark is likely true if we are discussing the value of pointless suffering but not if there is a teleological component to the suffering. Curiously enough, pro Kohl, a Christian need not advocate a principle of preserving life at the price of protecting needless, unredemptive suffering, but only the principle of preserving life at the price of protecting purposeful, redeemable suffering. The Christian, as I understand him, is not advocating pointless suffering, nor is he maintaining the thesis that mere physical life is always a good thing. The Christian seeks to minimize unredemptive human suffering, but he accords redemptive suffering all its rights in order to conquer it.

It is a truism that we all suffer at some time in life, if by "suffer" we mean undergo some form of pain or displeasure or mental anguish. We are all at one time hungry, annoyed, anxious, distressed, ill, nervous, etc. But perhaps the term "suffering" is more properly applied to periods of *intense* pain or displeasure or mental anguish, and the consequent frustration of some basic (nontrivial) human needs and goals. The concept of suffering includes the concept of pain, but not vice versa.

Is the proposition "prolonged suffering is evil" necessarily or contingently true? If we mean *instrumentally evil*, then the answer is clearly in the negative. If we mean *intrinsically evil*, Kierkegaard at least would again answer in the negative. Indeed he suggests that suffering is "blessed."

> If, however, someone comes along who with personal truth dares say: It is blessed to suffer, the world goes stark raving mad; nothing, nothing incites a world so much as this. For the fact that there are those who come to suffer—that is, against their will, and then find it anything but blessed to suffer—this the world is able to understand and have sympathy for, because this, after all, is how the world itself interprets enjoying life—since the one who suffers against his will and finds it an unhappy experience actually is a hedonist, in agreement with the world. But that "suffering is supposed to be blessed" is, after all, a shocking thing, says the world. It is mutiny against the world's whole theory of enjoyment.[6]

I am not sure if Kierkegaard held that suffering was intrinsically good. To deny that it is intrinsically evil, as he did, is not to affirm its intrinsic goodness. But it does seem clear that he thought some forms of suffering were instrumentally good.

In his *Purity of Heart*, Kierkegaard sets the stage for our investigation:

> Let us speak of a whole life of suffering or of some person whom nature, from the very outset, as we humans are tempted to say, wronged, someone who from birth was singled out by useless suffering: a burden to others; almost a burden to himself; and yes, what is worse, to be almost a born objection to the goodness of Providence.[7]

Since my focus is on suffering per se and not (at least directly) on the morality of infanticide, I need not get involved with the sticky linguistic issues raised by the latter term. For instance: is a thirty-year-old victim of cerebral palsy who requires constant nursing care not still a child, yet chronologically an adult? Also, we normally think of *infants* as very young children, roughly, age one day to seven years; but legally an infant is normally classified as any child who has not reached puberty, roughly, fourteen years for a boy, twelve for a girl. Perhaps the term *infanticide* in these discussions is often more appropriately defined as *childicide*.

JOHN DONNELLY

A good workable paradigm to keep in mind for the *indirect* applications of my discussion of suffering would be a case of spina bifida (meningomyelocele) suffered by a person roughly between the ages of five and twelve. Here the afflicted person is rationally aware of this greatly incapacitating malformation of his central nervous system, but his life expectancy is quite normal—given complex and expensive medical attention. (I am assuming that the risk of hydrocephalus has been checked by surgery, although there continues to be repeated and expensive pediatric, urological, and orthopedic treatment.) It is important that the afflicted person be rationally aware of his affliction, else he merely experiences pain but does not suffer. For example, a one-year-old child who is inflicted with Tay-Sachs disease in some sense does not suffer, although pain is felt. Suffering would seem to involve a rational awareness of pain and as a consequence the frustration of many of one's human life-projects.

Despite its "mutiny against the world's whole theory of enjoyment," Kierkegaard finds value in suffering. He writes: "There truly is a fellowship of suffering with God, a pact of tears, which is intrinsically very beautiful" [#4583]. Needless to demonstrate, our present age does not view suffering in such a sanguine, grandiose light. Paradoxically enough, Kierkegaard often writes as if people ought to so value suffering —even out of nonreligious motivations.

> It is well known that suffering and pain are a condition for many kinds of distinctiveness, such as with poets, artists, religious individualities, and the like. Without these sufferings they would not have become great. Take away their sufferings, give them an easy life, grant them what they desire— and it is all over with greatness. If they had their desire satisfied and the suffering taken away, they would lose even more: ergo, they ought to be happy in their suffering, so happy that they would not wish it removed. But then again they are beyond suffering. I wonder if an individual so situated could really understand this. [#4590]

In short, Kierkegaard is suggesting that the dismaying leads to the upbuilding, that suffering is a necessary condition for the moral/religious life. The turf of suffering provides virtue's breeding ground. As such it is to be welcomed. Nonetheless, Kierkegaard's encomium of suffering could still be viewed as primarily instrumental in design.

> Do you believe, then, that if you were thoroughly healthy you would easily or more easily achieve perfection? Just the opposite: then you would yield

easily to your passions, to pride if not to others, to an intensified self-esteem and the like. In that way sufferings, even though a burden, are a beneficial burden, like the braces used in the orthopedic institute. [#4637]

Kierkegaard proceeds to speak of "physical suffering, the infirm body, (as) a beneficial memento." Indeed, he offers the caveat to any planned worry-free, pain-free utopia, that "to be thoroughly healthy physically and mentally and then to lead a truly spiritual life—that no man can do" [#4637]. I think the *cannot* here is at least that of physical impossibility, and that Kierkegaard is not indulging in what appears to be somewhat characteristic hyperbole. He is saying, I believe insightfully, that the spiritual life (either a distinctly religious one or a nonreligious life of moral integrity) involves essentially a love for and commitment to the virtues, and that such a pursuit of virtue in a hostile environment is bound to tax the mental and physical strength of even a healthy individual. (Kierkegaard reminds us indirectly that medicine is as much a *caring* science as it is a *curing* one.) The spiritual life, Kierkegaard suggests, involves an initiation into suffering "by inward conflicts, by fear and trembling, by trepidation, by anguish of soul, by agony of spirit, being tried besides that by all the sufferings which are more commonly talked of in the world. A witness to the truth is a man who in poverty witnesses to the truth—in poverty, in lowliness, in abasement, and so is unappreciated, hated, abhorred, and then derided, insulted, mocked. . . ."[8]

But such utilitarian justifications or uses of suffering are not entirely to Kierkegaard's liking. The value of suffering transcends the rationale of the second stage on life's way. "The purely human conception of suffering can never go further than *either* to interpret suffering as ultimately teleological (one suffers for a time, a certain number of years, etc., in order to achieve this or that or become this or that, etc.) *or*, if the suffering continues, then to bear it patiently, but it is an evil" [#4681]. As Kierkegaard reminds us so often—one must go further!

Kierkegaard contrasts the "secular mentality" with the Christian view on suffering. The secular mentality relates to a higher goal out of a profit motive, but this inverts the fundamental relationship "for when the lower relates to the higher in order to profit from the relation, then the lower is actually higher than the higher from which one wishes to profit" [#4696]. By contrast, in the essentially Christian view, one favors relishing suffering in an *active* way and not just suffering passively or patiently. Hence Kierkegaard is recommending that a Christian choose suffering. "The best would be that you yourself voluntarily be inexhaustibly imaginative in inventing means of torturing yourself, but should you not be that strong—assuming that there is some truth in you, that you hate yourself—then you dare hope that God will have mercy on you and help you to come to suffer" [#4711]. Of course, a congenitally afflicted child does not choose to suffer in the sense that he can freely will his illness, but he and those who care for him might freely choose to accept it. Despite his often outlandish rhetoric, Kierkegaard is offering us no deontology of suffering, for one is not choosing suffering per se, but rather as a means "for discerning the witness of the Spirit" [#4692]. The former leads to a perverted masochism; the latter is truly liberating. Its justification, however, is theological and not philosophical. In the moral order suffering is tolerated principally because of its instrumental worth; in the religious order it is relished as a necessary condition of faithful witness.

From a religious perspective then, more specifically a Christian one, Kierkegaard is saying that the meaning of life is contained in suffering. Christendom, an inauthentic form of Christianity, has fostered the misleading idea that a Christian can acclaim the martyrs from afar and by this ersatz route have suffering eradicated from his life: "He has suffered and now the rest of us will have it easy" [#4711]. The all too common mistake here is to believe that Christianity is really nonrigorous,[9] and if it is not so *de facto* perceived, then this is due to those worldly forces or physical circumstances that have not permitted it to be so actualized. Kierkegaard claims Christendom offers a distorted conception of martyrdom, neglecting that "to be Christian is to be martyred" [#4711]. Again, Kierkegaard seems to be suggesting not that human life is intrinsically good so much as that suffering is not intrinsically bad. He is reminding us that the periphery of the Christian's itinerary is that of the cross.

Unhappily, Kierkegaard contends, Christendom has managed to soften the view that suffering is blessed by its "blasphemous pandering" [#4626]. *Pace* the "born-again" surrogates of today, Kierkegaard would insightfully suggest that such phenomena of revitalization are but signs of this misplaced doctrine. Kierkegaard, the master of irony, would take sardonic delight at the recent issues of *The Humanist* that rebut the current revitalization of religion in American life. The humanists fail to recognize that what they perceive to be a religious fervor is in fact just the opposite. Christendom is not their antagonist; but Christianity is. "What harm has been done to Christianity by taking mildness all by itself—and men have thereby been fooled into the fancy that they are Christians and Christianity has thereby been unmanned—instead of taking rigorousness along with it and gaining fewer but more genuine adherents" [#4642]. Having made this easy accomodation with the secular, Kierkegaard finds it not at all surprising that so-called Christians are not persecuted today on a large scale. Christianity, Kierkegaard avers, has become excessively *propositional*—a Christian is a person who accepts certain doctrines or intellectually assents to certain statements of belief. Instead, Kierkegaard favors a nonpropositional view, a mode of existing *qua* Christian, an imitation of Christ. He writes: "A doctrine does not inconvenience, does not excite and arouse persecution" [#4661]. That is, self-renunciation as a doctrine does not embarrass or invite persecution, but as a behavior pattern it is just the reverse. Unfortunately Kierkegaard's fondness for *aut-aut* gets the better of him here—the two accounts are perfectly compatible (and essential to true Christianity), and the practical strength of the latter is girded on the theoretical foundations of the former.

Yet, while Christianity is represented by Kierkegaard as "suffering truth" [#4649], it is also modeled on the life of Christ, and so, joyful.

> It teaches that there is enormous suffering, but that this enormous suffering nevertheless is light—not so light that it means that there is no suffering, no, light, although it is equally true that the suffering is enormous, consequently at one and the same time: enormous suffering—and yet light. [#4647][10]

Here we have a paradox, more apparent than real! Suffering is the price of God's love.[11] "Christianity clearly considers suffering to be the mark of the God-relationship: if you do not suffer, you do not have anything to do with God" [#4681]. It is true, as Kierkegaard avers, that "if you are not willing to suffer, you will then be free from God's love" [#4688], but somewhat questionable whether "the closer to God the more suffering" [#4698]. I say "somewhat questionable" (for obviously an eight-year-old child suffering from advanced spina bifida could reject belief in God, or if a believer, need not have suffered that physical affliction to be close to God), but I am not convinced it is false that proximity to God involves at least intense psychological suffering as an essential component of that voluntary *imitatio Dei*. Indeed, it would seem to be the case that however prosperous the external conditions of a Christian's life may be, those who deliberately imitate Christ love virtue and hate vice, and in a perfidious world, are bound to suffer *inwardly* at the apparent triumph of evil. But, unlike Ivan in *The Brothers Karamazov*, they do not "hasten to return the ticket" they've been sent. As a consequence of his gospel of suffering, those in charge of afflicted children should not commiserate with them or bemoan their affliction but instead suffer with them;[12] nor should the afflicted child seek to arouse such lament in his guardians.

Despite how guilty the world may make them appear, physically afflicted children are innocent. And innocence is a rare (and precious) commodity in a world increasingly devoid of it, and too often hostile to it. For a Christian, any instance of suffering innocence takes on increased significance as a reminder of Christ. The great moral imperative of the Christian remains that direct punishment of the innocent is wrong. Such a principle is quite consistent with the precept of mercy and certain active/passive forms of euthanasia. The Christian need not hold that, *pace* Anscombe, *one ought never wilfully (actively or passively) kill an innocent person*, only, *one ought never wilfully (actively or passively) punish an innocent person*. It requires considerable effort to prove that all instances of killing are instances of punishment. It also requires considerable argument to show that all instances of suffering involve instances of punishment. With the current debate about the morality of infanticide, those Christians, who in hindsight longed to be in Israel in the time of Pilate, now have their chance, however vicariously.

Notes

1. O. Ruth Russell, *Freedom to Die: Moral and Legal Aspects of Euthanasia* (New York: Dell Publishing Co., 1976), p. 225.

2. This presupposition is criticized in my "Suicide: Some Epistemological Considerations," in *Analysis and Metaphysics*, ed. Keith Lehrer (Dordrecht: D. Reidel Publishing Co., 1975), and my forthcoming "Suicide and Rationality," in *Language, Metaphysics and Death* (New York: Fordham University Press, 1978).

3. H. Tristram Engelhardt, Jr., "Ethical Issues in Aiding the Death of Young Children," in *Beneficent Euthanasia*, ed. Marvin Kohl (Buffalo, N.Y.: Prometheus Books, 1975), pp. 183-184.

4. I might add that I would not choose either of these illnesses as paradigms for discussions on the morality of infanticide. Apart from the usual difficulties involved in discussions on whether it is moral to kill, such ailments pose added complications as the inherited blood disorder, sickle cell anemia, principally affects blacks, and raises complicated issues of racism and genocide; and cystic fibrosis principally affects the lung and digestive tracts of whites.

5. "Voluntary Beneficent Euthanasia," in Kohl, *Beneficent Euthanasia*, p. 137.

6. *Soren Kierkegaard's Journals and Papers*, ed. Howard V. Hong and Edna H. Hong, vol. 4 (Bloomington: Indiana University Press, 1975), #4583. Subsequent references to this volume will be placed in brackets within the text.

7. Soren Kierkegaard, *Purity of Heart*, trans. Douglas V. Steere (New York: Harper and Row, 1956), p. 160. Kierkegaard did not specifically address the topic of the morality of infanticide.

8. *Kierkegaard's Attack Upon Christendom*, trans. W. Lowrie (Princeton: Princeton University Press, 1946), p. 7.

9. Cf. Kierkegaard on "spoonerisms," #3837.

10. "What good news? Not: here is money, here is health, here is status, etc.—no, no, then it is no longer Christianity. No, for the poor the gospel is the good news that to be unfortunate in this world (in such a way that one is abandoned by human sympathy, and the worldly zest for life even cruelly tries to make one's misfortune into guilt) is a sign of the God-relationship . . ." [#4685].

11. Cf. #4688.

12. Cf. #4716.

Karen Metzler

If There's Life,
Make It Worth Living

The quality of life for an infant born with a birth defect is established long before its conception. Society's attitudes toward diseased, disabled, or disfigured individuals mirror its attitudes toward life and death. Many social and environmental factors that influence individual action and feeling grow from the initial confrontation between one person and another person who is handicapped. Infanticide for those afflicted with a severe handicap is the ultimate negative reaction; it results from other less dramatic but still debilitating actions against persons that are handicapped: prejudice and discrimination in education, employment, daily activities, and personal relationships.

The psychosocial circumstances surrounding the birth of a defective infant relate directly to the issues of death and dying. In birth and death, one is confronted with questions concerning the meaning and value of human life.

A newborn's injured condition reminds us of human vulnerability, the ultimate realization of which is death. Society, through its individual members, may wish for the death of the imperfect infant: it is a biological mistake, which those perceiving it wish they could erase.

The desire for the death of an imperfect infant may persist even when there is a good prognosis for survival or intellectual development. Death becomes desirable as a means of escaping suffering for the infant;

however, the suffering continues on the part of the parents and society, and the form it takes is the realization of failure.

If an infant born with a birth defect should survive, he still represents a failure to realize the ideals of perfection and perfectability. In a society that idealizes and idolizes the body beautiful, athletic achievement, mental development, and upward mobility, a person who is handicapped threatens the sense of security of those who encounter him, because he is supposedly unable to attain what society considers success and a good life (an "inability" reinforced by prejudice and discrimination).

Those persons who are most doubtful about their own ability to meet societal standards tend to compare others as well to the social demands for success and acceptance. They often become the persons who reject the handicapped individual the most; yet all, even the most secure and mature, sigh in relief that they are not handicapped and hope it never happens to them, although disability is always possible in human life.

Attitudes and assumptions about these handicapped individuals were propagated through fears, fantasies, and misinformation, instead of knowledge and fact. The lack of personal contact, due primarily to the limited opportunities for participation in society's mainstream, caused barriers of prejudice to be built against persons who are handicapped. Society's basic attitudes toward the handicapped emerged: if they were acknowledged as persons, they were objects of curiosity; if their painful difference caused a hesitant awareness of their condition, they became objects of fear.

This fear often leads to the rejection and isolation of a birth-defected infant. Even from the time of its birth, parents may refuse to take the child home with them, and, if he is taken home, he is a statistically greater risk for neglect and abuse than are normal children. Parental response to their child establishes his psychosocial life and can determine the quality of the infant's future.

The mother-infant bond, the infant's first attachment to and relationship with another person, is based largely on physical contact, and an infant's physical attractiveness influences his desirability and affects the mother's ease in contact with him. If the infant has medical complications, the mother may be reluctant to touch and hold the child, even after being given permission by attending medical personnel. Nonattachment between mother and infant may occur even in the presence of nonvisible disabilities, such as in the instances of cardiac difficulties. Emotional withdrawal by parents who do not otherwise abandon their child may result from fear that the infant will die, a fear based on the physical and medical realities facing the child.

The child itself is born into a preexisting family unit that has developed its own interpersonal dynamics and history. An infant who is handicapped becomes an added stress on the members of each family. While a couple may have expected to become parents, neither have been prepared for the responsibilities of dealing with a handicapped child. With the development of amniocentesis parents could gain additional time to prime themselves emotionally for a birth-defected infant but, confronted with the unanticipated reality of the birth of a defective child, the parents will react in a manner consistent with their own personalities and their own experiences with illness and disability.

The basis of parental response is grounded in the prevailing social attitudes and assumptions about those persons who are handicapped, to which is added the parents' own personal reactions of guilt and anger at bringing a defective child into the world. The handicapped child as a biological entity does not determine the responses of his parents or others in general, but his birth places the event within a psychosocial context.

For example, the child of a young couple has been born with a cleft lip. The mother had a brother with the same defect, but the new father, with no prior experience of illness or handicaps, was left emotionally devastated at the baby's birth. As a counter-example, another couple, who, throughout childhood experienced positive encounters with retarded individuals, were more able to accept their child who was born with Down's syndrome.

Although grandparents and extended family members may be inaccessible, due to the mobility and frequent relocation of today's society, they also influence parental response and acceptance of a birth-defected child. The parents of the child may feel that his imperfections have caused them to be seen as failures in the eyes of their parents. Extended family members, grandparents, and the parents themselves may feel frustrated in their new roles; the child's condition negates the realization of their hopes and plans for him, particularly if he is a first-born child. Then, if the infant remains an only child, the fulfillment of the parents' various emotional needs that are related to their offspring becomes equally frustrated.

Other children in the family must also incorporate the birth-defected infant into their own personal development and lifestyles. They must cede expectations of perfection for the infant and be supported and prepared for the effects their handicapped sibling will have on them as individuals, and on the family as a whole. Further disruptions in family routines, should the birth-defected newborn require further hospitalization, must be anticipated and dealt with, and the other children need more reassurance, as they learn to cope with strained family resources of money, time, and attention.

Society reacts to the infant on the basis of his handicap and the family is similarly stigmatized. In facing such stigmatization, the parents' response to their newborn child who is handicapped establishes the foundation for the reactions of their other children, their families, and their friends. The normal developmental needs of all the children must be considered; so, the child that is handicapped must neither consume all of his parents' time and attention, nor become the scapegoat for family problems not necessarily related to him and his handicap.

The success with which the other family members deal with their individual feelings, the feelings of others within the family group, and the feelings of the handicapped child himself determines how effectively the child is welcomed and accepted as a natural part of the family. To achieve these goals, and to assure that the infant has as normal a childhood as possible, family counseling and contact with other families having children with similar problems are often beneficial in maximizing the quality of the later life of the child who is handicapped.

A constant feature in the life of a handicapped individual, and one that also influences his normal development, is the frequent contact with a myriad of medical personnel. Doctors, nurses, and other health-related professionals are also people, and they experience the same natural feelings that other human beings do when confronting an individual who is handicapped. The initial feelings of discomfort, shock, anger, denial, and depression, common to everyone, may be worked through by all and result in feelings of acceptance and compassion.

The significant and crucial difference between the reactions of medical personnel and the reactions of other societal members to a person who is handicapped is that health-related professionals have made a deliberate personal decision to enter a field where they encounter disease, disability, and disfigurement daily. Too often, however, particularly in dealing with a birth-defected infant, medical personnel avoid contact with the handicapped individual and his family, in an attempt to protect themselves from experiencing the natural human feeling of discomfort.

In addition, the medical profession's role-model is that of "healer," which carries the implied responsibility of "curing" the patient. However, in instances of chronic illness and disability and birth defects, a total and perfect cure may be unobtainable in terms of the current level of medical technology, knowledge, and skill. In such cases, medical personnel should emphasize the comforting and compassionate aspects of their professional roles, instead of stressing the curative role, in their care of their patient.

Intellectual understanding and knowledge are not all that is sufficient to enable medical personnel to react easily and supportively toward those persons who are handicapped. The experience and awareness of one's own gut-level feelings, even those deemed socially unacceptable, and the recognition that medical personnel are not exempt from experiencing such negative feelings gradually lead to the ability to see beyond the handicap and into the human being.

The natural feelings of helplessness and hopelessness that surface first at the birth of a defective infant may prompt others to avoid both the child and his family, just when emotional support is vital. If the infant should die, either naturally or as a result of withholding life-supportive measures, medical personnel should not terminate their involvement with the family. Instead, they should offer follow-up counseling and support to the family.

Some persons, in order to avoid the extensive demands of a habilitation program for the infant, suggest infanticide in those few cases where such a choice exists. The ultimate denial and rejection of the newborn implicit in infanticide does not free its advocates from the emotional impact of disease, disability, and disfigurement.

At some point in life, all persons encounter the handicapped, no matter how brief or superficial their contact might be. Attention and effort should be directed toward the development of society's ability and capacity to acknowledge uncomfortable feelings, in order to increase the potential for acceptance of and comfort with handicapped persons. Compassionate and understanding encounters with those who are disabled foster the movement toward greater integration and participation of handicapped individuals in the mainstream of society.

There is neither a guarantee that any human being will be born free of disease, disability, or disfigurement, nor any assurance that one will remain unimpaired throughout his life. A five-year-old, normal at birth, may be struck by a car and left paralyzed; a teen-ager may be permanently injured in a diving accident. Many healthy, able-bodied young men, doing military service for their country, may return as disabled veterans to face the social conditions that limit the handicapped. Cancer victims, even those cured or in remission, are denied insurance and employment opportunities because of the persistence of other people's fears that they may be "tainted," or that cancer necessarily results in an untimely death. Burn victims endure the inability to be freely mobile and visible in the community, because of others' reactions to seeing them.

Many defects are not immediately noticeable at birth. Cerebral palsy, epilepsy, deafness, birth traumata such as a lack of oxygen affect the child's later development. Then too, there is the inescapable reality that thousands of children, healthy at birth, are destined to become battered children, the victims of emotional and physical abuse that may sometimes result in permanent disability or death.

Individuals afflicted with any of these conditions are as subject to social negativity and frequent medical interventions as the infant born with a noticeable birth defect. Since persons with facial disfigurements are the least accepted social group, and since any impairment is usually linked with mental retardation, despite the fact that most handicaps neither impair social function nor impede intellectual development, it becomes apparent that the mere existence of a handicap, whatever its cause, elicits prejudice and negative social response.

The possibility of a being afflicted with a handicapping condition from a variety of causes remains a reality for persons of all ages. For some handicaps, there are cures at the present time; others are not medically remediable. Handicaps must be seen within their social context: while the medical model focuses strictly on an isolated individual and his physical symptoms, a more holistic view of handicapping conditions is necessary. Because designations such as *normal* or *exceptional* are socially defined and determined, persons who have been successfully rehabilitated from a medical standpoint still retain the social stigma of being handicapped; thus, they still encounter prejudice in the form of reduced opportunities, educational neglect, and vocational and interpersonal rejection.

The concept of normalcy needs to be revised so that it no longer negates the personhood of the individual. Exceptionality should refer only to a child's developmental rate, rather than to his whole being. The birth-defected infant becomes an exceptional child that has developmental needs and a rate of development beyond the minimum standard range designated by society as a comparative measurement of its children's progress. This definition of exceptionality allows a child to be ahead of, behind, above, or below the social norm.

The norm and the direction of deviation from it remain the standard criteria by which society evaluates its members. Persons of recognized achievements, talents, or genius differ from the average American, but, since they symbolize the actualization of man's potential, they are desired and revered by society. The handicapped, however, symbolize human vulnerability and limitation, and they differ from social norms in a negative manner. Were they socially recognized as contributors to the general welfare, they would be valued in a positive frame of reference.

Society perceives handicaps as negative qualities, and so disease, disability, and/or disfigurement become socially unacceptable; thus, the handicapped individuals are subjected to fear, denial, avoidance, and pity when they confront society.

The fear experienced in encounters with the disabled reminds individuals of their personal vulnerability, and challenges their ability to successfully cope with a handicap within the context of their own lifestyle. Attitudes and actions that reflect a lack of awareness of the special needs of the handicapped indicate denial. Avoidance is demonstrated when the handicapped person is shunned as a partner, friend, employee, or mate; its extreme manifestation is segregation for the handicapped in institutions isolated from the mainstream of society. When fund-raising campaigns feature poster children or other handicapped individuals, their appearance and disabilities evoke pity. Society's members respond with monetary contributions or token material kindnesses but not human companionship.

The poor societal conditions that exist for the individuals who are handicapped in our society should not determine whether birth-defected infants are allowed to live or die. The excessive medical expenses, social stigmatization and isolation, limited educational opportunities, and unemployment or underemployment that face the handicapped are manmade social problems that need to be redressed for all individuals who are affected, instead of being denied or avoided in those instances where a choice of life or death is possible.

While the quality-of-life for handicapped children and adults can be improved, their presence in our society emphasizes the need for responsivity and flexibility in meeting the requirements of all its members. The community should assist the handicapped individual and his family in integrating their handicaps into their daily lives, and society should provide the handicapped with opportunities to fully develop their potential.

The array of different opportunities for development makes us unique from each other; but the denial of opportunity can limit the quality of life. People are what we make of them and what we help them make of themselves.

At the time of birth we are not aware of what the future holds for an infant. Necessary changes effected by society could result in a more equitable quality of life for all handicapped persons. However, the real issues are not merely the infant's ability to have a "quality life" and an awareness of future capabilities, but rather the need for a social reappraisal of what qualities should be a part of human experience and the concomitant acceptance of the handicapped in the mainstream of society.

Joseph Margolis

Human Life: Its Worth and Bringing It to an End

When is life no longer worthwhile, no longer worth living?

The question is compelling but tasteless. It's compelling because our technology presses us to consider new possibilities and newer dreadful actualities that move us to cry, enough. It's tasteless because, reflecting on these and the ancestral condition of man, the question becomes demoralizing: it's unanswerable after all by any familiar inquiry. The prospects of nuclear calamity, the Sahel drought, the apparent hopelessness of Bangladesh, the exhaustion and disorganization of natural resources, the rise in pollution, the increased incipience of early cancers, the inevitability of global triage, and a thousand imminent such disasters force us to question even the point of planetary survival. Still, turning with whatever humanity to the plight of the spina bifida infant, the fetus conceived out of incestuous rape by some already seriously defective but sexually precocious child, elderly inmates of neglected institutional homes contemplating the likelihood and meaning of irreversible senility, the double, prophetic threat of the Quinlan case—that we may survive at some drastically reduced level of existence through a pure fluke, or worse, through an unbidden intervention—turning to consider such contingencies, we may well fail to attend to the subtleties of the question. For, regarding the fetus, the infant, the senile and the incompetent, the comatose, the unreflecting and the instantly suggestible, the unintelligent, the distracted, as well as the future and as yet nonexistent, we cannot even pose the question to those our humanity insists we must consider. As for ourselves, we are embarrassed at once by the possibility of responsible suicide, euthanasia at the hands of those who love us, the cool institution of the living will, intermediary medical strategies that permit us to view the imminence of death produced without apparent responsibility, as well as by our doubts regarding the competence and authority of others to answer the question decisively and effectively in our own case. Nor is this all. For it is terribly easy to confuse the question's resolution in one kind of case with its resolution in another.

Consider that the practice of capital punishment does not require that the life of an executed man be worthless, no longer worth living. Capital punishment imposes its penalty in spite of contingent possibilities every bit as attractive as those that fall to one's own executioner. And the surgeon who, by a skillful, even undetectable reflex, prevents the birth of a potentially viable but monstrously deformed life, calls into play a maxim of some sort that assigns to that life a counterfactual rationality: he thinks that if the fetus were to choose to live or die, it would—perhaps like me or like any rational being similarly confronted—favor not coming into the world at all. It is impossible, therefore, considering such cases, that we should fail to appreciate the extraordinary delicacy of attempting to answer the initial question.

We answer it largely by modifying it till it becomes manageable, and by introducing distinctions that relieve us of the fear of being utterly misunderstood. For there is no question that is more serious than the question of when, with respect to ourselves or others—it being in our power to choose—to end or authorize the ending of a life or to preclude or authorize precluding the conception of life, on the grounds that the life or possible life in question is not or would not be worth living or worth enough to live.

One line of distinction is particularly helpful. It does not actually address the issue, but it anticipates irrelevancies. First of all, we must sort out talk of future and as yet nonexistent persons from talk of potential and as yet not actual persons; secondly, we must sort out talk of actual, competent persons from talk of potential persons or of incompetent, perhaps even former persons. The point is this. No moral reflection of any serious degree whatsoever can fail to consider the interests, the needs, the rights of future generations, or obligations due them. But there *are* no such generations. On the other hand, the key setting in which to raise our initial question concerns when precisely *we* ourselves, acting reflexively, are prepared to end our own lives or to honor the decisions of one another. Related judgments and decisions regarding the incompetent fetus and the other functionally incompetent persons already mentioned, can only be conceptually parasitic on just these decisions and judgments. So it may well be—or at least it may well be conceded—that fetuses for instance are not or are not yet persons, as a number of theories have maintained;[1] but the concession is *utterly* irrelevant to the resolution of our question, once the question is pertinently posed with regard to *them*.

The upshot is that our question cannot possibly be posed in the same way for the would-be members of future but nonexistent generations and for the actual members of classes of creatures linked in a biologically unique respect to actual persons, whether or not the latter are themselves viewed as persons (potential, defective, former, or otherwise characterized). It may well be that one cannot answer the question regarding a fetus or infant in precisely the same way in which one answers it for oneself and for other competent persons; but the question *has* point, cannot be dismissed, cannot fairly be treated as a technical or merely instrumental question, a question of convenience or of merely biographical interest—where, on some theory, *actual* nonpersons of the relevantly unique sort are involved. Put in the most straightforward way possible, we can never suppose that life is (on any view) *no longer* worthwhile or worth living where the quality of lives of future generations is concerned. It *is* a moral matter to affect the quality of such lives, but there is no sense, continuous with the sense in which we claim to justify ending our own lives, in which we may end the lives of the nonexistent. Where there is no beginning—in the mortal world at least—there is no end. On the other hand, there is just such a continuous sense bearing on the ending of the lives of fetuses or of the senile, *whether or not* we choose to call these creatures persons any longer. Our question may have to be altered, but it can never be dismissed as morally irrelevant. There is an essential difference between "possible," nonexistent persons and actual creatures, linked by one line of potentiality or another, leading from or leading to actual persons.[2]

The relevant conceptual connections are now fairly obvious. Questions regarding how we may alter or affect the lives or the quality of the lives of possible future generations concern only the consistency of our *own* policies regarding provisions *we* make for the quality or term of life of all actual persons, in particular, provisions bearing on the management of certain strategic facilities and material conditions. Talk about future generations is, in effect, talk about the intentions of actual generations. But questions regarding how we may alter or affect the lives or the quality of the lives of potential or former or defective persons, of creatures uniquely continuous with actual persons, concern the responsibility of affecting the lives of *actual creatures*. Both are morally relevant sorts of questions. But the first *does not concern any creatures at all*—except ourselves, whereas the second concerns creatures in some important respect other than ourselves. We simply have no *relationship* to future generations, though, as morally responsible agents, we must contemplate such relationships: failure to do so is simply failure to be in touch with the human condition. But we have an actual relationship with actual creatures uniquely linked with the class of actually competent persons: failure to address the management of this relationship as a morally relevant matter is, at bottom, failure to grasp the scope or extension of morally pertinent relationships. So it makes no difference whether we treat fetuses or infants or the senile or the others already mentioned as persons: for, if they are persons, they are defective or incompetent or not yet competent persons; and if they are not persons, they are creatures uniquely continuous with those that are persons, and they exemplify a condition that obtains universally, viz., that we all develop from fetuses and all risk incompetences of the various indicated sorts.

This shows at a stroke the silliness of trying to decide whether to end the life of a fetus or infant or senile or comatose creature merely *by* pronouncing that the creature in question is not a person. For, either the pronouncement labels the antecedent judgment that we may justifiably end the life of this or that creature, or else it does not affect in the least the eligibility of our question. But of course, to say so is to say as well that, as promised, the distinction so far drawn is no more than tangential or preliminary to the original issue. We do not yet know how to decide when life is no longer worth living: we have confirmed only that it is an entirely fair question, one way or another, regarding creatures that are deficient or not yet fully competent in the way in which those that can pose and settle the question for themselves may be said to be competent. Hence, too, we see that it is the judgment and behavior of the latter that are central to the entire matter.

Once we concede these distinctions, we see as well that, if our question is at all eligible, then it could not be a contradiction to maintain that the life *of a person* is not worth living or not worth living any longer. *A fortiori*, our question would be eligible for creatures that, as persons, are deficient or defective or merely potential in one way or another. This leads us inexorably to qualify the original question. For there is something grossly mistaken about the presumption that if the life of a person may justifiably be ended—one's own or another's—then it can only be because that life is not or is no longer *worth living*. It is not in the least inconceivable that a worthy or worthwhile life, a life still worthy or worthwhile, may justifiably be ended precisely in order to close that life in the most favorable way, under terms thought suitably congruent with just such merit or quality.[3] Otherwise, natural death itself proves to be a puzzle: for, to treat death as signifying that some preceding life had ceased to be worth living—simply because it was now ended—flies in the face of the unrealized possibilities of a life cut short; and to treat it as compatible with some preceding life's having had significant worth, however unrealized, opens the possibility of deliberately cutting life short without denying the worth of living or of living further. For instance, a man who has lived a rich life may, in order (so he supposes) to avoid the horrible later stages of some incipient disease, elect to end his own life *now*. There is no reason in the world why he must suppose (i) that his life up to this moment or at this moment was not or is not worth living; or (ii) that his life passing beyond the present moment could not or probably would not continue to be worth living; or even (iii) that his life through the last stages of his disease might not still be worth living. There is simply *no* conceptual difficulty in maintaining both that one's own life has value, is worth living, or that life is worth living, or that the lives of others are worth living *and* that it makes rational sense, believing that, to end one's life *now* or even to favor ending another's life. All that is required is that one supposes, reasonably enough, (a) that we are all mortal creatures; (b) that ending one's life, rationally, is no more than assigning by one's own hand the determinate limit of one's inherent, determinable mortality; and (c) that one does so for appropriate reasons. There have been all sorts of arguments designed to show that one *never* has the right to end one's own life or that one could never rationally justify doing so. But *every* argument of that sort is either question begging or based on an antecedent tenet that is itself not open to relevant challenge. Biblically based injunctions and analogous charges based on an alleged dependence on some variously personified Nature demonstrate the point.[4] To hold either that God or Nature has "given" us our lives, so that we cannot deliberately "take" them is simply to subscribe to a doctrine that—however admirable and persuasive—*is incapable of independent confirmation*. That is the essential point. For, granting it, we see at once that it is hopeless to prove—in a way open to any sort of objective discovery, as if the point and worth of human life or of particular lives could be found by an inquiry rather similar to whatever would be needed to determine the tolerance of a bridge—that it is quite all right now to end my own life or to take or approve the taking of another's life. To disqualify the argument from revelation or the inspection of Nature's purpose is to refuse to take the question, "*When* is life no longer worthwhile?" in that literal sense in which an assignable interval of time may be confirmed as the *correct* interval *for the species*. There is no such discovery to be made. But that means that the justification for ending one's own life or the life of another, whether person or suitably related creature, can only be formulated in terms of the convictions and experience of the *interested* parties. There is no neutral way to decide the matter: we act here only as partisans, that is, *as* interested parties; the best we may hope for is that we act as reasonable or rational partisans.

In effect, this is a simple and powerful argument. Grant that we are mortal, grant that we are rational, grant that there is no way to discover or confirm that we are forbidden to end our lives or that there is an appropriate natural time for doing so, grant that ending one's life is not inherently irrational. If this much be conceded, then it is quite impossible to assess the defensibility of ending one's life, except in terms of personal conviction, personal history, and the experience of the race regarding the conditions of sustained interest in living. No one can adopt a purely disinterested view about his own intention to end his life; and, under the circumstances, no one can suppose that such an intention is illegitimate, merely as such. So there are at least two points to be pressed here: (i) that, though we are interested in when and how we shall die, there is no way of discovering the appropriate moment either for the species or for individual persons; (ii) that to favor ending one's own life or another's does not entail that the affected life is not worth living or utterly lacks value. It is enough that the issue enlists our attention as rational agents and that one's continuing to live or to let live may be judged not preferable to death.

The argument, of course, is an ellipsis. What it signifies is that man's moral concerns are directed, at least minimally, to the management of his prudential interests—the preservation of life, the reduction of pain, the gratification of desire, security of person and property, and the like—which themselves *presuppose*, both reflexively and regarding others, a continuing *interest* in living on.[5] Hence, those moral concerns cannot enforce such an interest, *a fortiori* an obligation, merely *to* live on. That's why suicide—and by extension euthanasia, infanticide, and abortion of certain sorts—troubles our conventional practice: they challenge the very presumption of a continued or implicit interest in living on; but they need not challenge the worth of living. There's no question that moral complications enter at once as soon as one agent, "acting in the interests of another," acts to end another's life; suicide is *sui generis*. But whatever those complications may be, their resolution cannot preclude the mere *eligibility* of ending another's life for cause or reason. Capital punishment, defensive wars, extreme measures in self-defense demonstrate that point at least. How much more obvious, therefore, that, lacking as we do any way of discovering when nature forbids or permits us to end our lives, we note that others, acting as rational agents, may wish to enlist us to end their lives or to help to end them or to allow them to end.

The fussiness of these last three distinctions suggests a potential dodge. John Lorber, for instance, a well-known British physician, who has apparently studied over a thousand spina bifida infants treated at Sheffield, favors a set of medical criteria for determining when or when not to treat a candidate baby.[6] Robert Reid reports that, on the application of Lorber's criteria to a group of thirty-seven children, twenty-five were not treated because of the severity of their condition. Regarding these:

> The infants were given all proper nursing care and appropriate food. Parents could take their children home if they wished. Beyond that, however, they were given no treatment; if they became infected by disease of any kind, they were not treated with antibiotics.
>
> Three of the children were dead within a few days, eighteen within three months, and all twenty-five within nine months.[7]

Nevertheless, as Reid observes, Lorber "was, and is, an opponent of euthanasia."[8] Now, it *may* be fair to distinguish euthanasia from the medical act of allowing spina bifida infants to die. But that has nothing to do with the fact that, acting rationally and knowledgeably, Lorber took responsibility for *bringing about the death* of those infants. Also, *if* it was morally defensible to bring those deaths about, then it must surely be an open question whether it would not also (or even more convincingly) have been defensible to take those lives in whatever active way would constitute euthanasia (though, of course, the law is opposed). Reid makes the pertinent observation: "The state of affairs is clearly ironical, and verges on the hypocritical. If a designated aim of medicine is that a child should die, why would it not be more humane to make it die?"[9]

The issue bears on the notorious question of Double Effect.[10] What we may say is this. If an agent acts intentionally to produce effect A, knowing that effect B is certain or so probable as to be practically certain, then the agent acts with the intention of bringing effect B about—even if, by some nicety of language, we concede that he did not act intentionally to produce effect B. The issue is the same in the setting of high altitude bombing (which cannot distinguish between combatants and civilians), the usual forms of abortion, and the withholding of medical treatment from spina bifida infants.[11] The point is that Lorber, however humane his intentions, must have made a decision to the effect that, whatever the worth of life, it was not sufficient to override the advisability of letting those twenty-five infants die. No fiddling with the dubious facilities of the Principle of Double Effect could make the slightest difference in that regard, however much it might protect the physician from the legal implications of euthanasia, and however pertinent it may be where the anticipated effect is believed to be significantly uncertain.

We have, then, sketched arguments for the following: (a) that ending the lives of creatures uniquely continuous with full-fledged persons is morally serious; (b) that acting to end the lives of such creatures (potential, defective, former persons) is fundamentally different from acting to affect the lives of future (nonexistent) persons; (c) that the reasoning that serves to justify ending the lives of such creatures must be conceptually parasitic on the justification for ending the lives of competent persons (ourselves or others); (d) that there is no way of discovering by any familiar independent inquiry whether we are forbidden to end life or when it is correct to end life, apart from our own sensibilities and interests; (e) that we are, as rational agents, interested in certain characteristic prudential concerns, in knowing when and how we are to die, and in judging whether it is better to die or to live on; (f) that judging that it is better to die rather than to live on does not entail that life is not worthwhile or no longer worth living or worthless; (g) that intentionally bringing about the end of a life is (perhaps) the genus of such determinate forms of acting as suicide, murder, euthanasia, and the like. We may add another consideration: (h) that so acting must rest on moral criteria that cannot be reduced to or replaced by technical criteria of any sort. This, of course, points to the complexity and easy temptation, for instance, of Lorber's putative medical criteria for deciding for or against the treatment of spina bifida babies. The question is identical with the question raised by the Harvard definition of brain death.[12] The issue concerns the morality of medical advice and cannot be displaced even by the admission that the parents of spina bifida children are expected to make the final decision. The point is that Lorber advises parents that, in his opinion, babies who meet one or more of his criteria for extreme forms of spina bifida should not be treated. There is no question that these criteria are humanely motivated and informed, and there need be no dispute about their being entirely reasonable; physicians who urge an alternative set of criteria are caught in precisely the same predicament: they cannot presume to settle the ethical issue on the basis of their medical competence.[13]

From here, it is but a step to understanding the rationale of ending the life of creatures uniquely continuous with persons, that are defective persons or only potential persons or potentially quite seriously defective or potentially incompetent persons—or of bringing about their death. There are, clearly, those who believe that the worth of life is such that no person may justifiably end or bring about the end of his own or another's life, as by suicide, murder, abortion, euthanasia, the denial or refusal of medical assistance, or the like. There are anomalies and dilemmas, of course. One has only to think of ectopic pregnancy, pregnancy due to incestuous rape, pregnancy that threatens the mother's life for contingent reasons, threats to the lives of Siamese twins of unequal viability,[14] severely deformed and defective infants that can survive only under enormous expense to parents capable of having normal children, religious sanctions against lifesaving intervention,[15] and it is obvious: (i) that very nearly everyone admits the defensibility of at least *some* exceptions favoring ending the lives of fetuses and infants and even full-fledged persons; and (ii) those who favor bringing about the death of creatures or persons of these sorts characteristically do so in a reasonably humane spirit. Related exceptions are even more abundant at the other pole of life, since, as we approach death, we are drawn to consider that ending one's life or refusing to prolong one's life may readily count as the rational decision of an agent facing the inevitable—in order, precisely, to insure some suitable congruence between the close of life and the worth one assigns (as a decidedly interested party) to that very life.

Once these considerations be admitted, it is impossible to mount a compelling argument against all forms of bringing about the death of those creatures, incompetent for a variety of reasons, that are uniquely continuous with persons. For, if they are capable of functioning as defective or fully competent persons, under conditons of extraordinary treatment (severe spina bifida cases) or even on occasion under conditions of ordinary medical care (cases of incestuous rape), we must suppose that they would judge (if they could) in accord with the sensibilities of competent, normal persons. For example, the onus of living in a family as the incestuous offspring of one's own grandfather might well be so horrible as to offset irretrievably whatever worth life itself possessed; certainly, perceived thus in advance, it could hardly be said that bringing about the death of the fetus could not possibly be either reasonable or merciful. Similarly the concern of competent adults to plan to end their lives or to allow them to end before their decline passes beyond a point that they themselves would regard as the limit of acceptability, as no longer congruent with their own sense of worth, provides us with a variety of models in terms of which to review, counterfactually, the judgment of severely malformed or defective fetuses or young infants.

Whatever the reasonable safeguards against abuse, whatever the dangers of the slippery slope, the mere moral eligibility of considering bringing about the death of incompetent creatures cannot be either precluded or viewed as marginal. On the contrary, the refinement of our various technologies forces the problem on us; for (i) we face the alarmingly difficult, potentially disastrous task of feeding and caring for the world's growing population at a time of dwindling material and financial resources; (ii) we have become increasingly capable of supporting life that is more and more marginally viable and less and less capable of full-fledged development as a person; (iii) we have become more and more certain, as far as the short run is concerned, of the precise disabilities fetuses and infants would have to face if permitted to survive; (iv) we know that it becomes increasingly difficult to bring to an end the lives of incompetent creatures, once they are permitted to draw the sustained affections of caring parents; and (v) the financial and material resources required for the care of these dependent creatures threaten to ruin the independent capacity of otherwise competent adults actually to care for them under realistic conditions and threaten to drain the resources of any of the usual supporting communities. In a word, the very same considerations that weigh on the minds of competent adults regarding the quality of life they favor for themselves—that lead them to consider suicide, euthanasia, the rejection of extraordinary means for sustaining life, and the like—weigh on communities (and are fairly weighed by them). Hence, since incompetent creatures are incompetent, we judge for them in the counterfactual sense that we suppose they would judge as rational adults of normal sensibilities would. It is in this sense that the decision to bring to an end the lives of selected fetuses and infants (also, the comatose, the senile, and others of the various sorts of incompetence mentioned) is *conceptually parasitic* on the decision of the competent to end their own lives or to bring them to an end. What the most reasonable grounds are for such decisions and what the best safeguards against abuse may be are difficult but subsidiary questions. What needs to be established first—the point of the foregoing remarks—is that it is entirely morally eligible to raise the question, that alternative policies may be more or less reasonable, and that the grounds for such policies depend on the prevailing sensibilities of adult persons, including sensibilities regarding the assignment of parental or other authority for the care of, and for limiting the care of, different sorts of incompetents.

Judgments regarding the lives of future generations and the lives of incompetent creatures are, therefore, dependent for different reasons on our judgments about our own lives: regarding the first, because it is only in terms of our own intentions that we concern ourselves with future generations; regarding the second, because their unique relationship to full-fledged persons obliges us, for conceptual reasons, to treat their "interests" as congruent or identical with our own.

Notes

1. Cf., for instance, Judith Jarvis Thomson, "A Defense of Abortion," *Philosophy and Public Affairs* 1 (1971): 47-66; and Michael Tooley, "Abortion and Infanticide," *Philosophy and Public Affairs* 2 (1972): 37-65.

2. Cf. Derek Parfit, "Rights, Interests, and Possible People," in *Moral Problems in Medicine*, ed. Samuel Gorovitz et al. (Englewood Cliffs, N.J.: Prentice-Hall, 1976). The argument is effectively directed against R. M. Hare, "Survival of the Weakest," in Gorovitz, *Moral Problems*.

3. See, for example, the cases that R. F. Holland considers, apart from his own assessment, "Suicide," in *Talk of God. Royal Institute of Philosophy Lectures (1967-1968)*, vol. 2 (London: Macmillan, 1969).

4. Cf. Immanuel Kant, *Lectures on Ethics*, trans. Louis Infield (New York: Harper and Row, 1963), pp. 147-154; cited in Gorovitz, *Moral Problems*; also, Leonard J. Weber, *Who Shall Live?* (New York: Paulist Press, 1976).

5. Cf. Joseph Margolis, *Negativities: The Limits of Life* (Columbus: Charles Merrill, 1976).

6. Robert Reid, "Spina Bifida: The Fate of the Untreated," *The Hastings Center Report* 7 (August 1977): 16-19. Cf. also, John Lorber, "Results of Treatment of Myelomeningocele," *Developmental Medicine and Child Neurology* 13 (1971): 279-303; "Selective Treatment of Myelomeningocele: To Treat or Not to Treat?" *Pediatrics* 53 (1974): 307-308; "Early Results of Selective Treatment of Spina Bifida Cystica," *British Medical Journal* 4 (1973): 201-204; and Robert M. Veatch, "The Technical Criteria Fallacy," *The Hastings Center Report* 7 (August 1977): 15-16.

7. Reid, "Spina Bifida," pp. 16-19.

8. Ibid.

9. Ibid.

10. Cf. "Double Effect, Principle of," *New Catholic Encyclopedia*, vol. 4 (New York: McGraw-Hill, 1967), pp. 1020-1022.

11. Cf. John Ford, "The Morality of Obliteration Bombing," *Theological Studies* 5 (1944): 261-309; Philippa Foot, "The Problem of Abortion and the Doctrine of the Double Effect," *Oxford Review* 5 (1967): 5-15.

12. Cf. Ad Hoc Committee of the Harvard Medical School to Examine the Definition of Brain Death, "A Definition of Irreversible Coma," *Journal of the American Medical Association* 205 (1968): 337-340; Robert M. Veatch, *Death, Dying, and the Biological Revolution* (New Haven: Yale University Press, 1976); Joseph Margolis, *Negativities*, ch. 2.

13. Cf. Joseph Margolis, *Psychotherapy and Morality* (New York: Random House, 1966).

14. A case of Siamese twins joined at the heart was recently reported in the *Philadelphia Inquirer*, Sunday, October 16, 1977. One headline in the extended treatment of the case—debated in advance by the parents, physicians, and several rabbis—was titled: "One must die so one can live."

15. Cf. the papers on Paternalism, in Gorovitz, *Moral Problems*.

Stephen Nathanson

Nihilism, Reason, and the Value of Life

I

What is the value of life? How do we assess life's value? Is the value of life something intrinsic, so that any life is valuable? Or is life's value conditional, so that in circumstances of one sort or another a life might have no value whatsoever?

These are difficult questions, which we may raise simply because we feel reflective, or which may be pressed upon us by the need to make "life-and-death" decisions. In the context of bioethical debates, it is assumed that life is generally precious, and it is the extreme value that life usually has which generates the intensity of debate, since intellectual conclusions may well influence the way life is treated.

There is another point of view, however, according to which life in general has no value at all. It is this bleak but intriguing view that I wish to consider here, in the hope that such an examination will help to clarify the value that life does have.

I shall begin by quoting passages from two novels by John Barth. The first is an argument that Todd Andrews, the main character of *The Floating Opera*, records in his journal on the night before he attempts to kill himself.

I. Nothing has intrinsic value.

II. The reasons for which people attribute value to things are always ultimately irrational.

III. There is, therefore, no ultimate "reason" for valuing anything.[1]

Waking the next morning, he adds the words "including life" to proposition III.

The second comes from *The End of the Road.* The character Jacob Horner is describing an experience of motivational paralysis that he had undergone. Describing how he had sat immobilized at the railroad station, he says,

> I simply ran out of motives, as a car runs out of gas. . . . There was no reason to do anything. My eyes . . . were sightless, gazing on eternity, fixed on ultimacy, and when that is the case there is no reason to do anything. . . . It is the malady *cosmopsis*, the cosmic point of view, that afflicted me.[2]

Neither Todd Andrews nor Jacob Horner meets death in these books. Todd's life is saved by an accidental slip in his suicide plan, and he goes on to see that if nothing has value, it is no better to kill oneself than to live. Jacob Horner is roused from his paralysis by the intervention of a self-styled psychotherapist and struggles against a relapse into paralysis. Both live, but neither is able to find any value in life.

Through his characters, Barth explores the interrelations between rationality and nihilism, and these passages express very directly a number of ideas which have played an important role in philosophical thought.[3] These are the following:

1. The real nature of things is that which is seen from a cosmic or ultimate perspective.
2. To view things rationally is to view them from the cosmic point of view.
3. When things are viewed rationally (i.e., from the cosmic point of view), they are seen to be lacking in value.
4. To attribute value to something is irrational.

This nihilistic argument is completely general and has nothing particular to do with life. Life is simply one of the many things that are seen to be lacking in value.[4] Yet, for some reason, the argument sounds more forceful when we are considering the value of life than it does in other contexts. We are seldom tempted to adopt the cosmic point of view when considering the value of the dollar or the value of a college education.

Yet, many otherwise practical people seem to think that the cosmic perspective is the appropriate one to adopt when evaluating life. Thus, it has frequently been held that the value of life is undermined if, for example, our souls do not live forever, or if the sun burns out some billions of years from now, or if our accomplishments are forgotten.

This point of view has been lucidly discussed and criticized by a number of writers, including Kurt Baier and Paul Edwards.[5] They remind us of some simple distinctions that are helpful in undermining the variety of metaphysical pessimism I have described. First, there is a distinction between Life as such and individual lives. Life, in its abstract singular form, applies to the totality of living things that either now exist, have existed, or will exist, and it is to be contrasted with the particular lives of particular individuals.

The second distinction is between two kinds of value or purpose. There is one notion of purpose, according to which something has a purpose or value if it fits into some overall cosmic scheme that applies to reality generally. In a second sense, something can be said to have purpose or value if it is useful in fulfilling the goals of particular agents.

With these distinctions in mind, we can now state more clearly the nihilist's view: Because Life has no cosmic purpose, individual lives have no purpose and hence no value. The value of individual lives depends on Life's having a cosmic purpose. But in what way does it follow that individual lives lack purpose and value if Life as such is without cosmic purpose? In one sense, this conclusion does follow, for if Life has no purpose because there is no overall scheme for it to serve, then individual lives will lack cosmic purpose because they will serve no overall scheme. What does not follow, however, is the claim that individuals cannot have aims and goals of their own that give their particular lives meaning and value. The absence of a cosmic purpose of either Life or individual lives does not translate directly into a lack of "terrestrial meaning" (to borrow Paul Edwards's term) for individual lives.

That the questions of cosmic and terrestrial purposes are quite separate is perhaps best brought out by assuming that there *is* some cosmic purpose to Life and seeing whether this guarantees that individual lives have purpose in some attractive sense. The answer is clearly negative. If the overall purpose of Life is, for example, to provide entertainment for a powerful malevolent demon, this would tend to undermine rather than enhance the status of individual lives. Indeed, the basic criterion for evaluating lives has to be a terrestrial one, for a cosmic purpose will only be life-enhancing if it coincides with purposes that individuals could adopt and pursue for themselves. As Edwards rightly concludes,

> If a superhuman being has a plan in which I am included, this fact will make (or help to make) my life meaningful in the terrestrial sense only if I know the plan and approve of it and of my place in it, so that working toward the realization of the plan gives direction to my actions.[6]

On this view, then, the cosmic perspective is seen either to be irrelevant to assessing the value of lives or to be subsidiary to terrestrial perspectives.

II

Why, then, is the attraction of the cosmic perspective so great? This question needs to be explored more fully if we are to succeed in exorcising the specter of cosmic meaninglessness. In what follows, I would like to suggest that the cosmic point of view arises from a distortion of a perspective that is important and appropriate, the rational point of view. It is no accident that both of Barth's characters could be described as exceedingly, even excessively, rational. They are driven to accept the appropriateness of the cosmic perspective by their understanding of what reason requires. What needs to be examined, then, is what I have labeled proposition #2 above: "To view things rationally is to view them from the cosmic point of view." Why are the rational point of view and the cosmic point of view thought to be identical?

I think we can understand this if we consider what we would be urging a person to do if we encouraged him to approach a particular subject rationally. One possibility is that we would be asking him to view it unemotionally. A person influenced by his fear of heights might judge that it was dangerous to be at the top of a tall building. In trying to convince him that there was no danger, we would ask that he put aside his fear for the moment and think about the tall barriers or heavy glass that prevent one from falling. We urge that he base his beliefs about the danger on the available facts rather than on his own aversion to heights. We get him to recognize the influence of features of himself (his emotions) on his view of the facts, so that he can try to discount this influence.

In this case, what we are doing is urging a person to overcome one of the many subjective factors that can influence belief. We are urging that he be *objective*. Although the emotions have long been seen as a hindrance to rationality by philosophers, they are not the only element to be overcome in striving for objectivity. We are aware of many respects in which our view of a matter is influenced by contingent features of ourselves or our situation. Each of us learns at a relatively early age that our spatial location is not the sole vantage point from which objects can be studied. Thus, we know that what appears to us to be small—by virtue of our own distance from the object—may in fact be quite large. Likewise, we come to see that what appeared to take up an exceedingly long time— because of boredom or anxiety—may well have consumed a short period of objective "clock time." There are, likewise, contingencies of background and upbringing that we urge a person to overcome in order to shed his prejudices or open himself to new tastes and experiences.

In short, when we urge people to be objective, we are urging them not to be influenced by the accidents of their nature or situation. We classify aspects of the world as real only if they would be recognized by a range of observers or knowers whose natures were quite different. Readers familiar with the problem of the reality of so-called secondary qualities (color, taste, smell, etc.) will recognize this criterion of reality. That which is to be considered the real nature of things must not depend on features of observers or perceptual conditions. Qualities that do depend on these are illusory or subjective.[7]

I think we can see now how the ideal of rationality leads to the attempt to achieve an objective perspective that is purified of all subjective influences. The best models for this perspective are from various realms of factual or scientific inquiry. Thus, for example, if we want to portray the location of an object, we draw a map or diagram that includes no reference to our own location. In physical theory, properties like color drop out of descriptions, and the properties which remain are, ideally, ones that would be recognized by anyone—ourselves, Martians, extragalactic creatures, even God. To talk about the cosmic point of view, then, is to talk about the view that any rational being could take, and what is known from that point of view has the status of the ultimately real.

In addition to the pressure toward the cosmic point of view, which is generated by an ideal of theoretical rationality, there is another related source that derives from the practical realm. In making decisions, we are sometimes led to act irrationally because we give priority to our present desires. The strength of felt desires overcomes our knowledge of long range interests or future desires. Prudence requires that we not give this priority to the present. It counsels that we overcome the undue influence of presently felt desires so that we can survey a longer stretch of our lives and rationally compare the value of objects presently desired to those that we expect to desire or need in the future. If we extend this common sense procedure and begin to view all of our needs and desires in the perspective of the long run, we may well fall victim to Jacob Horner's malady, "cosmopsis." The prudential view helps us to see that current, strongly felt desires may not in the long run be very important. The cosmic extension of the prudential point of view leads us to see that no matter what we choose, the end result will be the same—death.[8] And even if we think that our actions will continue to have effect beyond our deaths, there is the still longer point of view, which astronomy indicates will include the death of all creatures who inhabit the earth.

If this sketch provides a plausible diagnosis of the attractiveness of the cosmic point of view, then it shows that the tendency to evaluate life from this perspective is not simply a result of irrational moods or feelings. It is, among other things, the ideal of rationality itself, which calls upon us to put aside particular desires and aversions that we happen to have, and to see the world from the point of view of a being possessing only cognitive powers. When we do put ourselves into the position of a being without desires, aversions, goals, or preferences, a being who registers the properties of the world in its mind but is indifferent to them, then it seems that we will find no value properties among those that constitute objective reality. On the basis of this test, we would be led to Todd Andrew's conclusion that there is "no ultimate 'reason' for valuing anything."[9]

III

Having come this far, we must now ask whether we can reject the cosmic point of view and its apparent nihilistic implications without rejecting rationality. I shall try to show that the answer is "yes," that reason not only allows but indeed requires the rejection of this perspective.[10]

The first thing to note is that the cosmic perspective, as presented above, is simply irrelevant to the practical decisions and evaluations that we all confront. Whatever its aesthetic or metaphysical charms, it leaves out the very sorts of factors which generate practical problems and which must be considered in solving them. To take a trivial case: if I am faced with a choice between chocolate and vanilla ice cream, and if the cosmic point of view requires that I ignore tastes and preferences, it can certainly provide no guidance. Indeed, it would be *irrational* to adopt this point of view because the factors it leaves out are precisely those that need to be considered. To say that one should choose between the two flavors while ignoring considerations of taste and preference is to render the choice purely arbitrary and irrational.

Even this simple example illustrates, I think, that the rational point of view and the cosmic point of view do not coincide. Reason requires attention to just the facts that the cosmic perspective forbids us to consider. Misconstrued in the argument for adopting the cosmic perspective is the role of our desires, emotions, goals, etc., in rational decision making. Seeing these as subjective factors, which are opposed to reason, we are urged to ignore them. In fact, they provide the material upon which reason operates. We can acknowledge the importance of the noncognitive features of ourselves without forsaking objectivity and impartiality. When I choose chocolate over vanilla because I prefer chocolate, my choice is dictated not only by taste and felt desire, but also by adherence to the following rational principle: Given a choice between x and y in a situation where S prefers x to y, it is rational—all things being equal—for S to choose x. That is an impersonal principle of rational choice, which could be acknowledged by a being that was indifferent to both x and y! To recognize this principle, then, is in no way to express one's own nonrational preferences.

There are many principles of rational choice, which can be stated objectively and which do not presuppose that one share the affective responses of the person actually making a choice. Thus, for example, I can call a person's act irrational if he chooses it, if it is less likely to bring about the end he aims at than some other act, and if he knows that it is less likely to do so. Whether or not I share his preference for the end in question makes no difference to this judgment.

Taking the cosmic point of view seriously as a test for values leads one to overlook the difference between the following two questions:

(A) Would a purely rational being (a being possessing only cognitive powers) necessarily choose x over y?

(B) Would a rational being with such traits as particular goals, preferences, needs, or desires necessarily choose *x* over *y*?

Question A yields the nihilistic answer, for such a being is, by definition, indifferent to *x* and *y* and would have no basis for choosing between them. Question B, however, makes reference to the contingent features of the being making the choice and, hence, allows for judgments of rationality. It is irrational (except under special conditions) to thwart one's own goals, ignore one's own preferences, leave one's own needs unmet, or frustrate one's desires. We lose sight of this when we formulate our questions in terms of the cosmic point of view and the purely rational being, and as a result, we are led to the misconception that all values are irrational.

IV

In putting forward these claims, I have relied on an intuitive sense of what value and rationality are. The way in which I have linked these is, however, quite close to that which is assumed in the argument from *The Floating Opera*. Todd's formulation appears to presuppose that things have value if there is reason for valuing them. This sort of view has been made an explicit part of an analysis of value by John Rawls. In a chapter of *A Theory of Justice* entitled "Goodness as Rationality," Rawls argues that something is good if it is an object of rational choice.[11]

Unlike Barth's characters, however, Rawls emphasizes that rational choices and evaluations are made within a context, even when we do not always specify what that context is. As he says,

> The basic value judgments are those made from the standpoint of persons, given their interests, abilities and circumstances.[12]

Basic value judgments, then, are relative to persons, and we speak of something being good, rather than good for X, only when particular interests or circumstances are widely shared, when, for example, they are aspects of human nature.

If Rawls is correct, we make judgments of value by asking whether a given X would be a rational choice for someone in particular circumstances. He writes:

STEPHEN NATHANSON

> A is a good X for K (where K is some person) if and only if A has the prop-
> erties which it is rational for K to want in an X, given K's circumstances,
> abilities, and plan of life (his system of aims), and therefore in view of what
> he intends to do with an X. . . .[13]

As with the cosmic point of view, we are asked to evaluate from a position that is impersonal. However, the context is filled out sufficiently to
allow for choice.

An important problem for Rawls concerns the rationality of life
plans, since they define the context of evaluation. If a person's life plan
were irrational, that would carry over to his particular choices. Rawls
devotes a good deal of attention to characterizing what a rational life
plan is. I am not sure his account succeeds, but for present purposes I
will accept what he says, with its emphasis on the relativity of values to
individual life plans.[14] Given such an account, what can we say about the
value of life?

One thing that is clear is that, on this account, the value of life is not
unconditional. In the words of a quip which pleased William James, "It
depends on the liver."[15] A life that has properties that are rational for a
person with certain aims, etc., to want in his life will be a good life. A life
totally lacking in such properties will not be good; it will have no value.
Indeed, on this account, a life could have a negative value, could be (so
to speak) positively bad. In such cases, it might be rational for a person
to choose to end his existence.

This way of thinking certainly accords with widespread views about
the value of life. Even if one believes, for example, that suicide is *immoral*, one would be unlikely to say that a person was *irrational* to end
his life if all that was ahead was torture and suffering.[16] One could, in
fact, grant that a particular life was of no value, that suicide was a rational choice, and still maintain that a person had an obligation to continue living. So, granting Rawls's formula for nonmoral evaluation does
not by itself require any specific moral appraisal.

One could insist that the life of the person in such a case still had
value, even though the future was filled only with prospects for suffering. Such an argument would distinguish between the life of the person in
itself and the particular conditions under which the person would live.
The point would be that the conditions are evil, though the life itself is
still of value.[17]

Let us consider another case, which, though odd, has connections with actual instances. Suppose a person to be afflicted with "anhedonia," the inability to derive satisfaction from anything.[18] Such a person might well sink into a state of lethargy and indifference, which would lead us to say that he no longer possessed a life plan or system of aims at all. In such a case, even though the person might not be suffering, we might want to say that his life had no value. Lacking a system of aims, desires, and preferences, unable to derive satisfaction from living, such a person might well be indifferent to the choice between life and death. Given even the slightest motivation to end life, his act would not appear to be irrational. If we assume that the state of indifference is known to be permanent, then the person has no life plan that provides a context for the judgment that life is better than death. One is tempted to say that this person's life is of no value because there is nothing he wants to do with it.

I want to emphasize that in describing this case, I am *not* saying that reason *requires* ending one's life. Given this state of indifference, continued living is as rational a choice as an end to life. Reason allows either living or death and requires neither.[19]

Now this sort of case is especially interesting because it approximates certain features of cases in which a person is thought to be in a permanent coma, or in which an infant is born with such extraordinarily severe defects that it will never develop a life plan.[20] The person in a coma is difficult to describe, for (assuming that he had been living normally before his misfortune) he did have a life plan. Does that person still have a life plan? This is difficult to say. To have such a plan is a dispositional state that does not require constant activity. We do not lose our life plans when we sleep and regain them upon waking. On the other hand, this person never will waken, never will be active again. How can we talk about the persistence of aims, goals, and desires?

It may turn out that we need not answer the question whether persons in these situations have life plans. The distinction between the defective infant and the comatose adult *may not* be centrally important, since neither can pursue the fulfillment of aims or goals. Perhaps what we ought to do is to ask what a normal rational human being would prefer were he given a choice between death and one of these positions. Would a rational human being prefer life under these circumstances or death? We can circumvent the question about life plans by specifying that whatever life plan might be possessed, it will never be achieved, and no steps can be taken in an effort to achieve it.

Unfortunately, such a test will not provide a means for settling the controversies about such cases. The spirit of Rawls's discussion suggests that a rational being in question will take primarily prudential considerations into account, and this would imply that when a person reaches a point at which no personal interests can be served any longer, that person would choose death. Life is no longer of value for him, as it is no longer the vehicle for carrying out his plan. However, to restrict the range of allowable reasons to prudential concerns is to beg the question, for some rational persons might include among the components of their life plan such things as living in accordance with moral or religious proscriptions of voluntary death.[21] Hence, though incapable of deriving further satisfaction or benefit from life, they might regard continuation of life until its "natural" end as something of value. Since such continuation would be part of their life plan, it would satisfy Rawls's criterion for being valuable.

In other words, the split between those who favor and those who oppose various forms of suicide and euthanasia would reappear within the life plans of individuals so that there would not be a unique answer to the question: "What would a rational human being prefer in this circumstance, life or death?"

This conclusion has a relativist and subjectivist ring to it, and one might wonder how far it differs from the remarks quoted from *The Floating Opera*. Have I not reached the conclusion that life has value if value is attributed to it? And is this not the same as Todd Andrews's journal entry that "the reasons for which people attribute value to things are always ultimately irrational?"

The answer to this is "no." The value of life does turn out to be relative, since it is conditional on what other things persons happen to value and, indeed, on their evaluation of life itself. On the other hand, it is not "irrational" to attribute value to what one prefers. *That* one prefers something may be a brute fact, but given that it is preferred, it is rational for persons to value it.[22] To use a previous example: my flavor preferences may be brute facts of a nonrational sort, but my decision to act in accord with my preferences is not a brute fact of a nonrational sort.

There is, in addition, a further respect in which the value of life is objective, and this derives from the fact that one can be mistaken in one's evaluations of one's own life. For example, a person who is despondent because of his failure to reach a particular important goal may believe that his life has become worthless when, in fact, many other aims, which he still values, are available to him. Hence, his negative evaluation is mistaken, and ceasing to attribute value to his life would be irrational.

That such errors are possible shows that the view I have developed does not make evaluations of life totally subjective. I will not pursue any further the problem of mistaken evaluations, but some of the questions I have raised can only be answered if a catalogue of types of errors could be given. Of especial importance would be an account of cases in which positive value is mistakenly attributed to life. Are there such cases? Presumably, those who urge the propriety of the cosmic point of view for such evaluations believe that there are, but this basis for judgment has, I hope, been shown to be faulty. In addition, someone might argue that a person, with no prospects for an active life, who continues to value his life would be mistaken, would be, indeed, the victim of an irrational preference. While I think this view has some plausibility, I see no way to defend it, and the Rawlsian analysis of value which I have used appears to provide no basis for it.

V

Let me summarize the conclusion this essay has yielded. I began with questions concerning the value of life, the manner in which the value of life can be assessed, and the opposition between life as a conditional or intrinsic value. I tried to explain why people are often tempted to answer these questions from a "cosmic point of view" and why this perspective is inappropriate. The appropriate perspective must take into account many facts about a person that are left out when the cosmic perspective is adopted.

The attempt to view things from the perspective of persons in particular circumstances appears to give support to the view that the value of life is conditional, since it depends on a person's life plan. Paradoxically, however, it turns out that for persons with a certain sort of life plan, the value of life is an unconditional feature. That is, certain people would hold that the continuation of life has value even when conditions fail to be satisfied that other persons regard as necessary conditions of life's having a value. Hence, any attempt to use a formula for value, like that of Rawls, as a means of settling controversies concerning the choice of death, in situations where a person can make no choice for himself, appears doomed to failure.

The only way in which a Rawls-type test could settle the controversy would be if one side could demonstrate that the life plans of the opposition are irrational. That is, (a) if one could show that it is irrational to prefer to *end* one's own life when further activity is impossible, or (b) if one could show that it is irrational to prefer to *continue* one's life when further activity is impossible, then the matter would be resolved. I do not myself see how either of these positions could be established.

Notes

1. John Barth, *The Floating Opera*, rev. ed. (New York: Bantam Books, 1972), p. 218.
2. John Barth, *The End of the Road* (New York: Bantam Books, 1969), p. 74.
3. I have dealt with a number of these issues in two previous papers: "Nihilism, Reason and Death: Reflections on John Barth's *The Floating Opera*," forthcoming in *Analecta Husserliana,* vol. 10; and in "John Barth's Critique of Pure Reason," unpublished.
4. Cf. Barth, *The Floating Opera*, pp. 166-167.
5. Kurt Baier, *The Meaning of Life* (Canberra: Australian National University, 1957) and Paul Edwards, "Life, Meaning and Value Of," in Paul Edwards, ed., *The Encyclopedia of Philosophy* (New York: MacMillan and Company, 1967), vol. 4, pp. 467-477.
6. Edwards, *Encyclopedia of Philosophy*, p. 472. A similar point is made by W. D. Joske in "Philosophy and the Meaning of Life," *Australasian Journal of Philosophy* 52 (1974): 95.
7. The classic discussion of primary and secondary qualities is in Locke's *Essay Concerning Human Understanding*, Book II, ch. 8, although similar points are developed by Descartes. For the historical background to this, see E. A. Burtt, *The Metaphysical Foundations of Modern Science* (1924; reprint ed., Garden City, N.Y.: Doubleday & Company, 1954); on Locke's use of this distinction, see Maurice Mandelbaum, *Philosophy, Science and Sense Perception* (Baltimore: Johns Hopkins Press, 1964), ch. 1, and my "Locke's Uses of the Theory of Ideas," forthcoming in *The Personalist*, 1978.
8. For expressions of this view, see the discussion of Darrow and Tolstoy in Edwards, *Encyclopedia of Philosophy*, pp. 468-469.
9. Strictly speaking, this need not be correct. Many theists would claim that God views reality from a cosmic, yet benevolent, point of view. Even apart from theistic assumptions, Bertrand Russell once wrote, "The infinite part of our life . . . shines impartially like the diffused light on a cloudy sea . . . it gives love to all, not only to those who further the purposes of the self . . . its impartiality leads to truth in thought, justice in action, and universal love in feeling." Quoted from "The Essence of Religion," originally published in *The Hibbert Journal*, 1912, and reprinted in *The Basic Writings of Bertrand Russell*, ed. R. Egner and L. Dennon (New York: Simon and Schuster, 1961), p. 566.
10. The helpful distinction between what reason allows and what reason requires is made by Bernard Gert in *The Moral Rules* (New York: Harper and Row, 1973), pp. 23-24.
11. John Rawls, *A Theory of Justice* (Cambridge, Mass.: Harvard University Press, 1971), ch. 7.
12. Ibid., p. 401.
13. Ibid., p. 399.
14. As I indicate, I have my reservations about Rawls's view, and I regard my use of it as a partial test of his analysis. If his view is helpful in dealing with the problem of the value of life, that will provide some confirmation of it. In fairness to Rawls, I should note too that he might well have reservations about my applying his analysis to the value of life. Life is, in his view, one of the primary goods, and it is not clear whether the value of primary goods is derived in this way or whether it is of a more fundamental sort. Hence, it is *possible* that my use of his analysis is a misuse.

15. Quoted in "Is Life Worth Living?" first published in William James, *The Will to Believe and Other Essays in Popular Philosophy* (Magnolia, Me.: Peter Smith, n.d.) and reprinted in *Essays on Faith and Morals*, ed. R. B. Perry (Cleveland: Meridian Books, 1962), p. 3.

16. For a defense of the view that suicide can be both moral and rational under certain conditions, see R. B. Brandt, "The Morality and Rationality of Suicide," in *Moral Problems*, ed. J. Rachels (New York: Harper and Row, 1975), pp. 363-387.

17. A similar distinction is sometimes made by hedonists who defend the view that even sadistic pleasures have value, even though the conditions in which they occur are evil.

18. William James cites the French psychologist Ribot as the originator of the term in *The Varieties of Religious Experience* (New York: Collier Books, 1961), p. 127. See, too, R. B. Perry's chapter, "The Pathology of Interest" in *The General Theory of Value: Its Meaning and Basic Principles Construed in Terms of Interest* (Cambridge, Mass.: Harvard University Press, 1926), p. 567ff.

19. I take this to be an effective counter-example against part of the view developed by Bernard Gert, *Moral Rules*, pp. 30-33f. I discuss this point in detail in my "Nihilism, Reason and Death"; see note 3 above.

20. R. B. Brandt has argued that in such cases, death is not an injury and thus is not morally forbidden. See "A Moral Principle About Killing," in *Beneficent Euthanasia*, ed. Marvin Kohl (Buffalo, N.Y.: Prometheus Books, 1975), p. 109.

21. That the manner of one's death can be a part of one's preferred life plan (apart from questions of suffering) is made clear by Socrates' discussion in Plato *The Phaedo* 61D ff.

22. This principle, though broadly correct, is subject to important limitations. Within the Rawlsian scheme, we could note that the preference must be compatible with the general system of aims and goals that comprises a life plan. In addition, if Bernard Gert is correct, there are certain desires that are in and of themselves irrational, so that having these desires would provide a person with no reason for satisfying them. For Gert's view, see chapter 2 of *The Moral Rules* and his paper, "Irrational Desires," in *Human Nature and Politics*, ed. J. Chapman and R. Pennock (New York: New York University Press, 1977), pp. 286-291. The latter paper is a criticism of R. B. Brandt's "The Concept of Rationality in Ethical and Political Theory," which is printed in the same volume, pp. 263-279. See, too, Brandt's "Rational Desires," *Proceedings of the American Philosophical Association, 1970*, pp. 43-64.

Marvin Kohl

Voluntary Death and Meaningless Existence[1]

Those who assume that voluntary death is morally permissible may be divided into various classes, according to the view they take of the question, "What are the necessary conditions for making this decision?" I will content myself with discussing three typical views, views held by those who believe that, given certain circumstances, it is permissible or better to leave than to remain in this world. I shall briefly characterize and criticize each of these views and then proceed to more closely examine respective positions concerning the nature and implications of leading a meaningless life.

One further preliminary point. Though I wish to discuss rival theories of voluntary death with special focus on the problem of meaningless existence, I will not dwell on the argument advanced by the extreme nihilist who maintains that, because nothing has intrinsic value, life is meaningless and therefore must be ended.[2] I reject this argument because, first, it seems to confuse the problem of an individual's finding meaning for his life with the problem of finding the meaning or purpose of the universe. Purposes can only be assigned to sentient beings; and, therefore, one who does not believe there is sufficient evidence for holding that the world is governed by a sentient being can only recognize the individual purposes of separate men and animals. Second, even if men could be content with discovering the nature and not the so-called purpose of the universe, it is clear from the evidence that is in, that the history of mankind is, in greater part, a history of a struggle against the undesirable aspects of nature. And once we understand the nature of ideals, of which morality is a part, we realize that so long as man is free to aspire he will long for the better life—for what ought to be, and not for what merely is. Finally, it simply does not follow that if nothing is of intrinsic value nothing is of value. A preliminary to finding meaning in one's life is that of finding values worthy of cherishing. In spite of the difficulty of doing so, one can wisely choose. The fact that man must ultimately choose his values or ends, it seems to me, is rather cowardly grounds for necessarily spurning life.

I.

1. Among those who believe in the right to end their own lives, there are some who think as follows: The hastening of one's own death is essentially an exercise in and expression of human freedom. The individual wants to leave life and embrace death. The argument for doing so is a simple one. Since a man's life belongs to himself, he not only has a right to depart from this world, but he need not have a noble reason for doing so.

As Seneca observes:

> An expedition will be incomplete, if one stops halfway, or anywhere on this side of one's destination; but life is not incomplete if it is honorable. At whatever point you leave off living, provided you leave off nobly, your life is a whole. Often, however, one must leave bravely, and our reasons therefore need not be momentous; for neither are the reasons momentous which hold us here.[3]

Similarly, he maintains that

> Mere living is not a good, but living well. Accordingly, the wise man will live as long as he ought; not as long as he can. He will mark in what place, with whom, and how he is to conduct his existence, and what he is about to do. He always reflects concerning the quality, and not the quantity, of his life. As soon as there are many events in his life that give him trouble and disturb his peace of mind, he sets himself free. And this privilege is his, not

only when the crisis is upon him, but as soon as Fortune seems to be play-ing him false.[4]

Evidently Seneca and his followers recognize that there are degrees of having a quality life. They also recognize that some reasons for dying are better than others. But in the last analysis, any reason is sufficient as long as it is not the result of external coercion.[5]

What is there to be said against this view?

There is, to begin with, the charge that it is inadequate because it fails to distinguish between reasons based upon full information and reasons that are not. To put an end to a life because full information warrants saying that a particular and otherwise irremediable problem ex-ists is one thing. But to do so as soon as Fortune seems to be playing us false is another, and one that appears to be deeply problematic, if not ir-rational. Another cogent reason for rejecting this view, and one that I will discuss more fully in the concluding pages of this paper, is that it fails to adequately distinguish between expedient and preferable means of problem solving. Voluntary death may often be expedient, but it is certainly neither always preferable nor as preferable as the followers of Seneca would have us believe.

2. This theory is a sharp modification of the first. Direct suicide is prohibited but indirect is not. Morally, one may not directly intend to cause one's own death. That is to say, one may not perform an act that must lead to death. However, one can perform an action that has a high probability of death if there exists a very grave reason for the performance of the act, and if the good or end achieved is sanc-tioned by law. Hence it is not only permitted, but it is even a duty at times, to sacrifice one's life in order, for instance, to make a confession of faith; to aid the sick in time of epidemics, if one is entrusted with the care of souls; and to defend one's country in time of war. Given this venerable tradition it is also (but not only) lawful to expose one's life to danger in order to preserve chastity; to risk one's life in saving those who are exposed to danger of flood, fire, or other natural disaster; and for sailors to go down with their ship, or soldiers to be blown up with their fortress or transport, when the purpose is to injure the en-emy.[6]

The great strength of this position is that it does not vaguely refer to morally sanctioned ends that justify endangering one's life, but specifies what these ends are. It has the merit of allowing for certain kinds of heroism and martyrdom. As such, it allows for the kinds of risks, the taking of which seem to be required for the normal functioning of society. Nonetheless, this position has its share of difficulties, not the least important of which is that it prohibits the direct, voluntary ending of innocent life, no matter how awful be that life or how kindly be the proposed death. The major worry here is, why is it a kindly act or a charity, and therefore virtuous and sometimes obligatory, to lay down one's life in order to help others but never permissible to lay down one's life in order to help oneself?

3. This is our own theory, and one form of utilitarianism.[7] According to this view, man has both the prima facie right to life and to relinquish life. The right to life is generally conceived as the right to have the bare minimum one needs for continued life, whatever that may require, provided it does not violate anyone else's similar right; to have protection against unjust assault or interference with vital interests; and to seek redress if that prove necessary. Because this right is an unusually complex one, we often refer to its various parts: the right to subsistence, the right not to be killed, the right to vital health protection, and the right to self-defense. The right to relinquish life—or what is more dramatically called the right to die—is in part, the other side of the coin. It is the right, under proper conditions, to die how, when, and where we choose or would choose if we were capable of doing so. From this point of view the question is not: Do we want voluntary death or do we not? The question is: How much voluntary death—direct or otherwise—do we want to allow, and where and when and of what kind?

A partial answer to this question is to suggest that voluntary death may be the best thing when altruism calls, when death is imminent, or when irremediable suffering or other circumstances make one's life irrevocably meaningless. That is to say, a kindly rational society would permit more than indirect or altruistic suicide. It would also allow the voluntary death of those who are afflicted with an incurable disease (or injury) in its terminal stage and of those unfortunate human beings who lead irrevocably meaningless lives. I will not elaborate on the general question of the justification of suicide, which, it seems to me, has been eloquently and more than satisfactorily answered by Sidney Hook[8] and Richard Brandt.[9] I am content for the present to outline a minimally acceptable position concerning those who are terminally ill and to suggest the direction that perhaps ought to be taken concerning those who lead meaningless lives of a certain kind.

In the case of those afflicted with an incurable disease (or injury), which is judged by reliable second parties to be in its terminal state, a kindly rational society would seem to want the following policy:

(1) Within the limits established by the similar rights of others, there should be relief of pain, relief of suffering, provision for general care and concern, and respect for the patient's right to refuse treatment.

(2) When a terminally ill or injured individual has signed a "living will" or expressed, as a result of reflective judgment, the wish to die, he (or she) has the moral right—and ought to have the legal right—to refuse or discontinue medical treatment, especially the use of extraordinary means of life support.

(3) When such an individual gives free and fully informed consent that his life be terminated, a physician ought to be legally permitted to place at the patient's disposal medication that would end life swiftly and painlessly; and where the patient is not physically able to administer to these needs, a physician should be allowed to induce death, or permit it to occur.

(4) When such an individual, a person afflicted with incurable disease (or injury) in its terminal state, is also in a state of irreversible coma or is an infant, consent may be obtained indirectly from an authorized representative acting in the patient's behalf, provided that that consent is not contrary to the known preferences of the patient.

The question of nonterminal cases is more complex and much more difficult. It becomes even more complicated when we introduce the term 'meaningless life' and claim that there appears to be some extensional overlap between the actual right to relinquish life and that of having a meaningless life. Let us, therefore, begin with a characterization of the latter term.

In judging a span of life as being meaningful many of us seem to mean first, that during the period in question the individual has some overall dominant goal or goals that give direction to those parts of his total life pattern and circumstances that he thinks are important; second, that the individual believes there is some genuine possibility that he will attain these goals; third, that the having of the goal or goals is sufficient to thwart chronic depression or melancholy and, in more optimistic situations, adds a special zest to life. On this view, a span of life becomes devoid of meaning roughly when, or to the extent to which, an individual cannot possess goals or when, if he can and does have goals, he believes they are trivial or impossible to achieve.[10] This, I suggest, is how most people who have studied the claims of those who hold that their life is meaningless, or who have had the experience themselves, would be inclined to characterize these notions. They may differ as to the nuances; but they share the common conviction that meaningfulness is not a permanent state of being, and that the circumstances of our lives *and* the disposition of our character mainly determine the measure of the meaningfulness we enjoy.

It would seem then as if we might proceed and say that to end a life that is irrevocably and completely meaningless is a morally right act, because such a state of consciousness is intrinsically undesirable. But the question may naturally be asked, does it not then follow that it is permissible to end the lives of all such individuals merely because they lead completely meaningless lives? This raises an important worry but does not, I think, strike at the heart of the matter. For one may reply, that if it is right to do whatever may prevent or eliminate the occurrence of an intrinsically undesirable state, then this conclusion does indeed follow. What is objectionable here, of course, is the notion that it is right to do whatever may prevent or eliminate the occurrence of an intrinsically undesirable state. We, for example, may abhor ugliness and believe it intrinsically undesirable, but few would be inclined to say that one is completely free to destroy all ugly things.

An attempt may be made to develop a more adequate argument. Thus one might say: Since we do not injure human beings when we allow their lives to end or put them to death even if they cannot, or have failed to, state their preferences if they are living a completely meaningless life, if the state of affairs that warrants that judgment is irreparable and irreversible, and if there is no or insufficient evidence to indicate they would not accept the judgment that their lives are meaningless—and, since killing a person is not something that is prima facie wrong in itself, but is roughly wrong only if it is an injury of someone, it follows that the ending or allowing of the ending of the lives of human beings who lead such lives is not prima facie wrong.[11] If, in addition to these requirements, the act in question is a great kindness, then to the extent that it is and *ceteris paribus*, we should end or allow that life to end. Thus the merciful extinction of life is morally permissible and indeed mandatory where it is not an injury to anyone and where, and to the degree, it rests on one or more of our moral duties, especially the duty of beneficence.

MARVIN KOHL

II.

There are several plausible objections. Limiting ourselves, in the main, to the problem of having a meaningful life, let us start by considering the charge that the terms 'meaningful' and 'meaningless life' are intractably subjective and therefore form a weak basis for part of a theory supporting voluntary death. To be more precise, the objection is as follows: "We are told that a meaningless life is one in which it is no longer possible, in practice, for the individual in question to achieve any of the goals he holds to be nontrivial and important. So that there is an objective safeguard to this theory: namely, that once we know what a person's goals are we can proceed to determine whether or not they are, in fact, achievable. This, of course, may be difficult knowledge to obtain. However, the more formidable difficulties lie elsewhere. What if the goals held to be nontrivial are really trivial? Or, what if the opposite be the case? What if an individual has very high, perhaps unrealistic, expectations? For example, what if an excellent chess player—who wants to be chess champion and nothing more—cannot do so? Suppose he therefore finds life meaningless? Is he then not morally entitled to end his life and entitled to do so, strangely enough, because he selected unwise goals? In short, since a person's goals are notoriously subjective and this theory is based upon these preferences, the theory slips into an untenable form of subjectivism."

There are several strands of thought running through this objection. Let us start with the definition of the term 'meaningless life' and admit that the term will, indeed, apply to situations where an individual may have goals of dubious value or apply to other situations where an individual may have unrealistic expectations. I distinguish, however, between the process of coming to understand the meaning of a phrase and ethical education. The latter consists in strengthening certain desires and weakening others, quite a different process. We may want people to hold certain goals but not to hold others. That is, in the main, what moral education is all about. So that if we find individuals who have dubious or unrealistic goals we may wish, and in certain circumstances would have an obligation, to attempt to reeducate them. If an individual only wants to be the chess champion and cannot, we may, for example, encourage him to develop new interests.

Similarly I distinguish between the process of determining whether or not a phrase has truth conditions associated with it, and linguistic prescriptivism. The former, in our present connection, comes down to determining the extent to which truth conditions may be associated with the claim-type: "My life is irrevocably meaningless, because my goals are unattainable and irreplaceable." The latter consists in giving reasons and urging that we should use language in a new or different way. Thus, one may urge that we define 'meaningless life' as "one in which it is no longer possible, in practice, for the individual in question to achieve any of the goals we hold or he ought to hold as being important." Or one may claim, as many do, that while life may appear to be humanly meaningless, in reality it is never so.[12] Or, and perhaps the most interesting, one may suggest that life always "has" meaning because there is always the possibility that a person may detect and accept a new pattern for his own life.[13] But whatever may be the merits of these proposals, one thing is clear: they raise a logically distinct issue. To the extent one fails to recognize this and substitutes, without supporting argument, an alternative sense of 'meaningless life' in order to guarantee that it never, or almost never, can be the case that a human being can have a meaningless life, to that extent, one not only evades the issue here being raised, but begs the question.

It is evident that there is a further distinction between having a meaningless span of life and having an irrevocably meaningless life. In normal living there may be periods where Fortune has frowned or arrived too early, and where one finds oneself living a completely meaningless life. Time, patience, fortitude, and/or developing new and viable interests often heal this wound. So that in a normal life one is likely to pass through relatively or completely meaningless periods. There are, however, certain lives that are totally irrevocably meaningless, when an individual cannot possess, can no longer possess, or cannot achieve any goals *and* when one or more of these conditions are irreversible. Certain cases of irreparable brain damage, monolithic or anhedonic personality, permanent coma, and impending inevitable death are some examples.

It is important also, to distinguish between believing p and knowing p, where p is the proposition, "My life is irrevocably meaningless." Our aspiring chess champion may say and truly believe p, but from a moral point of view it seems necessary that he should also know p. That is to say, it seems necessary that he know, not only that he cannot be the chess champion, but that he cannot (presumably psychologically or morally cannot) develop other goals. But adequately to discuss the reasons for and against supposing that this is a necessary condition would take us far too long. And fortunately it is unnecessary for our present purpose, since the only question we need answer is whether or not there are objective constraints on making judgments of meaninglessness, and what some of them are. I conclude, then, that there is a difference, first, between the judgment that one is having a meaningless life, and second, between *believing* that one is leading an irrevocably meaningless life and *knowing* that that is the case, and that, to the extent a theory of voluntary death is not cognizant of these distinctions, it is quite untenable.

I now turn to the second, and final, objection I here wish to consider. It raises some large questions, and even though we cannot be fully justified either in accepting or rejecting the hypothesis, it is, I think, well worth considering what is at issue. The charge, usually leveled by advocates of the first theory, is, why hold the line against voluntary death to acts of rational altruism, imminent natural death, and irrevocably meaningless existence? Or to put this objection into more limited but sharper focus: When you are not living the good or the happy life, why should a benevolent society want to morally prohibit your exit when it is freely chosen? For is it not true, as Seneca suggests, that at whatever point you leave off living, provided you leave off nobly, your life is a whole?

This subject is so vast that it is impossible, within a limited space, to do more than outline some of its aspects. To be sure, the quality of the ending of a person's life seems to weigh much more heavily in the judgment of whether or not he has lived a happy life. That is to say, men are more inclined to judge a life that ends well to be a happy one than a life that ends poorly. But this is not to say that one who has ended life wretchedly, no one will or should call happy.

The question may be brought within manageable compass by distinguishing two radically different schools of thought. On the one hand, it is often suggested that, since the purpose of life is to experience or obtain some balance of enjoyment, creativity, or excellence, and since it takes time to achieve these goals, quantity of life is necessary, and the more important condition. On the other hand, we have Seneca and others claiming that it is not mere living that is a good but living well; that it is the quality, not the quantity of life, that really counts. Formulated in terms of these extreme positions, the question is, what is more important, quantity or quality of life?

My view is this: There is a difference between having a meaningful, a good, a happy, and a perfect or blessed life. A meaningful span of life seems to require that during the period in question the individual has some overall dominant, progressively obtainable goals that give direction to those parts of his total life pattern and circumstances that he thinks or is likely to come to think of as being important. A good life is one that, inspired by beneficence and guided by knowledge, achieves at least partial goals. Within this context it is commonly asserted that, aside from saints, lunatics, and men of genius, a man is happy if his basic needs and correlate interests are more than minimally being successfully met, and if he is generally pleased with and appreciative of that success. A perfect or blessed life, on the other hand, is one in which all rational desires are met. Each one of these levels seems to be necessary for the achievement of the next and higher level. So that neither the good, happy, nor the blessed life is possible without having a meaningful life.

By way of reply we can now say, at least in a rough and tentative sort of way, that if the good life requires the partial achievement of goals, among which are basic needs and correlate interests, then it seems obvious that quantity of life is a decisive factor. It is for this reason, I believe, that we are usually greatly pained by the death of children. We sense, among other things, that their lives are incomplete because they did not live long enough. Similarly, we often say of a person who dies in adolescence that he at least lived a good life. But often we add that, because he did not live long enough, he was not able to fully taste happiness. Another, perhaps clearer way of saying this, is that the phrase complete life is an elliptical way of saying completely meaningful, good, happy, or blessed life. And, since each level above that of meaningfulness usually requires time and progressively increasing amounts of time, quantity of life is usually a progressively increasing requirement of the good, happy, and blessed life. Thus, to the extent we rationally pursue these goals, we must take very seriously both the quality and quantity of life.

We are now in better position to understand why a beneficent society would not generally want its members to leave off living because they are not leading the good, the happy, or the blessed life. A beneficent society distinguishes between expedient and preferable means of problem solving. Suicide, for example, certainly is an expedient way of coping with failure to live the blessed life, but no rational man is likely to hold that it is always, if ever, the preferable solution. Similarly, few men doubt that death ends worldly unhappiness, but most, I suggest, would consider it the least preferable of workable means. This point is of more than theoretical interest. For the failure to make this distinction is a contributing factor in the rise of nonrational suicide, especially the suicide of adolescents. Stoic rhetoric aside, the dirtiest death is not always preferable to the daintiest slavery or failure. The ending of one's own life is not always the best means of achieving a given end.

A beneficent society will allow its members to leave off living, but only for good reasons and only where that death is the preferable solution. Where early death is the preferable moral solution there is an obligation to allow for a good death. A beneficent society, on the other hand, is not intoxicated with the idea of death. For it realizes that a good death is but a small part of a good life. But it is a natural part of the idea of a good life that life itself be laid down for a noble reason, or after the best that it can give has been fully enjoyed and death is imminent, or when life is so awful that it is merely a form of brute subsistence, totally devoid of quality. An ideally good life, in this sense, is like an ideal meal. A splendid meal that ends poorly is, as a whole, not a good meal. What most men desire is a splendid meal with a splendid dessert. Similarly what almost all men seek is as good a life in age as in youth. When both are not possible, wisdom demands that life should at least end well. For it renders a significant service to mankind and the practice of morality to know that, after having lived a relatively impoverished or wretched life, one does not have to end wretchedly. And while a good ending is not a substitute for a good life, the glories of beneficence require that those who have led lives of little enjoyment and much adversity at least should have the opportunity of leaving this world in the contrary manner.

Notes

1. An earlier version of this paper was presented at the *International Symposium on the Dying Human*, Tel Aviv, January 16, 1978.

2. An essentially similar argument is raised by Todd Andrews, the narrator and central character of John Barth's *Floating Opera* (New York: Bantam Books, 1972).

3. Seneca, *Ad Lucilium Epistulae Morales*, (Cambridge, Mass.: Harvard University Press, 1962), II, p. 171 (Epistle LXXVII).

4. Ibid., p. 59 (Epistle LXX).

5. For an excellent example of a Seneca-type contemporary libertarianism, see: Thomas S. Szasz, "The Ethics of Suicide," *The Antioch Review* 31:1 (1971), pp. 7-17.

6. This position is primarily associated with traditional Christian theism. See: Thomas Aquinas, *Summa Theologica* 2.2.64.5-7 especially St. Thomas's enjoinder that "moral acts take their species according to what is intended, and not according to what is beside the intention. . . ." (Seventh Article.) A position bereft of the element of blameworthiness, but otherwise similar, is described by Bonhoeffer. Thus, he writes that "in man the right to live must be safeguarded through freedom. It is therefore not an absolute right, but a right which is conditional upon freedom. The right to life has as its counterpart the freedom to

offer and to give one's life in sacrifice. In the sense of sacrifice, therefore, man possesses the liberty and the right to death, but only so long as his purpose in risking and surrendering his life is not the destruction of his life but the good for the sake of which he offers this sacrifice" (Dietrich Bonhoeffer, *Ethics* [New York: Macmillan, 1965], p. 166).

7. This particular form of utilitarianism would include those who hold (1) that the moral significance of our actions or rules depends upon their actual or probable consequences; (2) that since happiness is generally more preferable than misery, there is a duty of beneficence that, in part, holds that we are entitled to the actual assistance of others and that, where it is necessary (as in vital or basic problematic life situations) to help someone in distress, it is society's obligation to do so; and (3) that, although the exact hierarchy of duties is far from clear, beneficence appears to be the architectonic positive duty.

8. Sidney Hook, "The Ethics of Suicide," *The International Journal of Ethics* 37 (1927), pp. 173-88. Reprinted in *Beneficent Euthanasia*, ed. Marvin Kohl (Buffalo, New York: Prometheus Books, 1975), pp. 57-69.

9. Richard Brandt, "The Morality and Rationality of Suicide," in *A Handbook for the Study of Suicide*, ed. Seymour Perlin (New York: Oxford University Press, 1975), pp. 61-76.

10. Cf. Paul Edwards, "Life, Meaning and Value of," *The Encyclopedia of Philosophy*, Paul Edwards, Editor-in-Chief (New York: Macmillan & The Free Press, 1967), p. 473; W. D. Joske, "Philosophy and the Meaning of Life," *Australasian Journal of Philosophy* 52:2 (1974), pp. 93-104; and F. C. White, "The Meaning of Life," *Australasian Journal of Philosophy* 53:2 (1975), pp. 148-150.

11. For a fuller discussion of this notion of noninjury and other parts of this argument, see Marvin Kohl, "Karen Quinlan: Human Rights and Wrongful Killing," in *Bioethics and Human Rights: A Reader for Health Professionals*, ed. Elsie and Bertram Bandman (New York: Little, Brown, 1978), pp. 124-127.

12. R. C. Chalmers, "Christianity," in *The Meaning of Life in Five Great Religions*, ed. R. C. Chalmers and John A. Irving (Philadelphia: The Westminster Press, 1965), p. 83; Arthur J. Dyck, "An Alternative to the Ethic of Euthanasia," in *To Live and to Die: When, Why, and How*, ed. Robert H. Williams (New York: Springer-Verlag, 1973), pp. 106-107.

13. Karl Britton, *Philosophy and the Meaning of Life* (New York: Cambridge University Press, 1969), p. 189.

Great Britain:
The Infanticide Act of 1938

(1 & 2 Geo. 6 c. 36)

*An Act to repeal and re-enact with modifications the provisions of the
Infanticide Act, 1922*   [23rd June 1938]

Northern Ireland. This Act does not apply; see s. 2 (2), *post.*

1. Offence of infanticide

(1) Where a woman by any wilful act or omission causes the death of her
child being a child under the age of twelve months, but at the time of the
act or omission the balance of her mind was disturbed by reason of her
not having fully recovered from the effect of giving birth to the child or
by reason of the effect of lactation consequent upon the birth of the
child, then, notwithstanding that the circumstances were such that but
for this Act the offence would have amounted to murder, she shall be
guilty of felony, to wit of infanticide, and may for such offence be dealt
with and punished as if she had been guilty of the offence of manslaughter of the child.

(2) Where upon the trial of a woman for the murder of her child, being a child under the age of twelve months, the jury are of opinion that she by any wilful act or omission caused its death, but that at the time of the act or omission the balance of her mind was disturbed by reason of her not having fully recovered from the effect of giving birth to the child or by reason of the effect of lactation consequent upon the birth of the child, then the jury may, notwithstanding that the circumstances were such that but for the provisions of this Act they might have returned a verdict of murder, return in lieu thereof a verdict of infanticide.

(3) Nothing in this Act shall affect the power of the jury upon an indictment for the murder of a child to return a verdict of manslaughter, or a verdict of guilty but insane . . .

(4) (*Rep. by the Criminal Law Act* 1967, *s.* 10 (2) *and Sch.* 3, *Part III.*)

NOTES

The words omitted from sub-s. (3) were repealed by the Criminal Law Act 1967, s. 10 (2) and Sch. 3, Part III.

Wilful. "Wilfully" in the words of Lord Russell of Killowen in *R.* v. *Senior*, [1889] 1 Q.B. 283, at pp. 290, 291, "means that the act is done deliberately and intentionally, not by accident or inadvertence, but so that the mind of the person who does the act goes with it"; see also, in particular, *R.* v. *Walker* (1934), 24 Cr. pp. Rep. 117; *Eaton* v. *Cobb*, [1950] 1 All E.R. 1016; and *Arrowsmith* v. *Jenkins*, [1963] 2 Q.B. 561; [1963] 2 All E.R. 210; but see *Rice* v. *Connolly*, [1966] 2 K.B. 414; [1966] 2 All E.R. 649.

Child under the age of twelve months. The question whether the child was under the age of twelve months is for the jury to decide but the judge may hold that there is no evidence to go to the jury (cf. *R.* v. *O'Donoghue* (1927), 97 L.J.K.B. 303).

Felony. The distinctions between felony and misdemeanour were abolished, and the law and practice applying to misdemeanour were in general made applicable to all offences, by the Criminal Law Act 1967, s. 1, p. 552, *post.* See also, in particular, s. 12 (5) of that Act, p. 561, *post,* as to construction of existing enactments.

Punished as if . . . guilty of . . . manslaughter. Under the Offences against the Person Act 1861, s. 5, p. 151, *ante,* the punishment for manslaughter is imprisonment for life or for any shorter term. For power to fine, see the Criminal Law Act 1967, s. 7 (3), p. 559, *post.*

Guilty but insane. The verdict is now to be that the accused is not guilty by reason of insanity; see the Trial of Lunatics Act 1883, s. 2, as amended, p. 225, *ante.*

Alternative verdict. A person who is tried for infanticide may be found guilty of child destruction; see the Infant Life (Preservation) Act 1929, s. 2 (2), p. 305, *ante.*

Arval A. Morris[1]

Proposed Legislation[2]

AN ACT Relating to the administration of euthanasia to certain severely defective children suffering from an irremediable condition; creating new sections; and providing penalties.

BE IT ENACTED BY THE LEGISLATURE OF THE STATE OF____

NEW SECTION. Section 1. Authorization of euthanasia. Subject to the provisions of this Act it shall be lawful for a qualified physician, or his professional medical agent, as authorized by a qualified physician's written statement, to administer euthanasia to a qualified child for whom the child's parent or guardian previously has made a written declaration voluntarily requesting euthanasia for the qualified child and which declaration is lawfully in force at the time of administering euthanasia.

NEW SECTION. Sec. 2. Definitions. The definitions set forth in this section shall apply throughout this Act unless the context clearly requires otherwise.

(1) "Physician" means a registered medical practitioner legally licensed and qualified to practice medicine in this state.

(2) "Qualified physician" means the specific physician in charge who will either administer or authorize the administration of euthanasia and who previously has received written approval for this specific administration of euthanasia from at least five of seven members of a professional medical ethics committee of this state.

(3) "Professional medical ethics committee" means a committee

created pursuant to section 3 of this Act.

(4) "Euthanasia" means the painless and quick inducement of death and may be accomplished by removal of medical treatment, by positive act, or by any painless and quick means.

(5) "Qualified child" means any severely defective child under the age of eighteen years in respect of whom two physicians, one of them a medical specialist in the particular area in question, have certified in writing that the child clearly appears to them to be suffering from a severe, incurable, and irremediable condition.

(6) "Irremediable condition" means either (a) a serious physical illness, including serious genetic defects, serious birth defects, or other physical impairment, which is diagnosed as severe and incurable and which is expected to cause a child severe distress or pain and to render him incapable of the rational or functional existence needed to enjoy the most minimal amount of human goods necessary to constitute ordinary human life in its most minimal sense, or (b) a condition of brain or genetic damage or deterioration such that what would be a child's normal mental or genetic faculties are so severely and irreparably impaired to such an extent that the child has been rendered incapable of leading a rational existence.

(7) "Declaration" means a witnessed declaration in writing made by a qualified child's parents-to-be or parents or parent if the other parent is dead or unknown, or legal guardian, substantially in the form set forth in this Act.

NEW SECTION. Sec. 3. Professional medical ethics committee—Rules governing. (1) The director of the department of (Social and Health Services) of this state shall, in consultation with the medical association of physicians in this state, adopt rules for the selection and operation of professional medical ethics committees. There shall be a number of such committees sufficient to carry out the purposes of this Act.

(2) Each committee shall have seven members representing persons of diverse backgrounds and occupations, such as attorneys, social workers, theologians, and others, but in no event shall any committee have more than three physicians among its membership.

(3) The duties of the committee shall be to review the diagnoses of the two physicians who have examined a child and all individual circumstances of each child's specific case on its own merits solely as those merits relate to that child (except for fully known conditions or diseases,

for which as a category—such as anencephaly—there is no reasonably possible medical remedy and in which event the committee may establish a policy governing each category of condition or disease instead of dealing with each case within the category), and after considering all the individually pertinent dimensions—scientific, medical, ethical, and others—the committee shall determine whether the administration of euthanasia would be in the better interests and welfare of the child. The committee shall make this ultimate decision without consideration of, or reference to, the interests or welfare of any person or matter other than the highest individual welfare of the particular child in question.

(4) The director of the department of (Social and Health Services) of this state shall also promulgate rules for determining who may or may not sign a declaration by way of attestation, for regulating the care and custody of written declarations and of written approvals or disapprovals of professional medical ethics committees, for appointing, with their consent, hospital physicians having responsibility in relation to qualified children who are subject to euthanasia, and for the prescribing of any matter he may think fit for achieving the purposes of this Act.

NEW SECTION. Sec. 4. Declaration made in advance. Subject to the provisions of this Act, a declaration shall come into lawful force and effect immediately after having been executed and shall remain in lawful force and effect unless revoked.

NEW SECTION. Sec. 5. Mode of revocation. A declaration may be revoked at any time by destruction, by notice of cancellation shown on its face, or by any other clearly communicated act of revocation, effected, in any way, by the declarant or to his order.

NEW SECTION. Sec. 6. Duties and rights of physicians, nurses, and professional medical agents. (1) Before causing euthanasia to be administered to a qualified child, the physician in charge shall make sure (a) that a valid written declaration exists and (b) that a valid written approval of the professional medical ethics committee exists for the administration of euthanasia in the specific case, and if the physician should determine that the professional medical ethics committee or the parent's or guardian's motivation or desire for euthanasia is supplied by any reason, or combination of reasons, other than solely for the sake of the child, then the physician shall not cause euthanasia to be administered.

(2) Euthanasia shall be deemed to be administered by a physician if it is prescribed by the physician in charge and by his written order euthanasia is administered to a qualified child by the physician's professional

medical agent or nurse.

(3) No person shall be placed under any duty by this or any other Act or by contract or by any statutory or other legal requirement, to participate in any way in any aspect of treatment or euthanasia authorized by this Act to which such person has a conscientious objection.

NEW SECTION. Sec. 7. Protection for physicians, nurses, and professional medical agents. (1) A physician or a nurse or a physician's professional medical agent who, acting in good faith, causes euthanasia to be administered to a qualified child in accordance with what a reasonable person would believe to be a valid written declaration and a valid written approval by the relevant professional medical ethics committee shall not be guilty of any offense.

(2) Physicians, nurses, or physician's professional medical agents who have taken part in the lawful administration of euthanasia as set forth in this Act or in accordance with subsection (1) of this section shall be deemed not to be in breach or violation of any professional obligation, oath, or affirmation.

NEW SECTION. Sec. 8. Offenses. (1) It shall be an offense punishable on information or indictment by a sentence of life imprisonment for any person wilfully to conceal, destroy, falsify, alter, or forge a declaration with intent to create the false impression that a parent or guardian desires, or does not desire, euthanasia for his child; it shall equally be an offense punishable on information or indictment by a sentence of life imprisonment for any person wilfully to conceal, destroy, falsify, alter, or forge any document or writing with the intent to create the false impression that a professional medical ethics committee has approved, or has refused to approve, euthanasia in the case of any child; and it shall equally be an offense punishable on information or indictment by a sentence of life imprisonment for any person wilfully to conceal, destroy, falsify, alter, or forge any document or writing with the intent to create the false impression that the physician in charge has authorized a nurse or any other professional medical agent to administer euthanasia to any child.

(2) Any person signing a declaration or any document or writing indicating that a professional medical ethics committee has, or has not, approved euthanasia, and who signs by way of attestation and wilfully puts his signature to a statement that he knows to be false shall be deemed to have committed the crime of perjury and shall be subject to its punishments.

NEW SECTION. Sec. 9. Insurance policies. No policy of insurance that has been in force continuously for one year shall be vitiated or legally impaired in any way by the subsequent administration of euthanasia to the insured.

NEW SECTION. Sec. 10. Administration of drugs. To remove doubt it is hereby declared that a child suffering from an irremediable condition shall be entitled to the administration of whatever quantity of drugs that may be required to keep such child free of pain.

NEW SECTION. Sec. 11. Forms of declarations. Declarations required under this Act shall be made in substantially the following style.

FORM I

Declaration made_____ 19_____, by____
_____, guardian or parent(s) of_____
_____, a qualified child.
I (we) declare that I (we) voluntarily subscribe to the matters now set forth: It has been clearly determined that my (our) child, who is named above, is suffering from a severe, incurable, and irremediable condition, as defined by the Severely Defective Children's Euthanasia Act of 19_____, which condition has been clearly and fully explained to me (us), and it has been determined by five members of the professional medical ethics committee that it would be in the better interests of my (our) above-named child to have euthanasia, which committee decision has been clearly and fully explained to me (us). In light of the above, but exclusively on the basis of my (our) independent consideration and judgment of the question, and after consultation with others, and solely because I (we) deeply believe that euthanasia is in the better interests of my (our) above-named child, I (we) do hereby request and authorize the administration of euthanasia to_____ my (our) child, at the earliest convenient time and circumstance.

_____
Parent or Guardian

_____
Parent or Guardian

We testify that the above-named declarant(s) voluntarily signed this declaration in our presence, and appeared to us to appreciate its full significance. We do not know of any pressure being brought to bear upon the declarant(s) to make this declaration, and we believe it is made by his/her (their) own wish and solely on behalf of the better interests of his/her (their) above-named child. So far as we are aware, we are entitled to attest to this declaration, and we do not stand to benefit by the death of the above-named child.

_____   _____

Witness   Witness

FORM II

Declaration made_____ 19_____, by____
_____ and _____ who
are about to become parents.
After full discussion with my (our) attending physician, Dr._____
_____, I (we) believe myself (ourselves) to be fully informed about the forthcoming birth of my (our) child(ren) and recognize that occasionally children are born who have severe defects or irremediable conditions, as that latter term is defined in the Severely Defective Children's Euthanasia Act of 19_____, which defect or irremediable conditions disable newborn children from ever having the basic capabilities of enjoying the minimal goods that constitute a bare minimum of ordinary human life—an example of this type of newborn is one that is anencephalic. Because I (we) believe that it is in the better interests of severely defective newborns, such as anencephalic newborns referred to above not to survive, I (we) hereby request and authorize that if our child, or if any of our children now about to be born, should be anencephalic or clearly of any equally severe and equally disabling disease or condition as such diseases or conditions previously have been determined by the professional medical ethics committee, then no active steps should be taken by anyone, and in particular that no resuscitatory techniques should be used, to prolong the life or lives of my (our) child(ren) so afflicted or to

restore them or any one of them to consciousness.

_____   _____
Parent-to-be   Parent-to-be

We testify that the above-named declarant(s) voluntarily signed this declaration in our presence and appeared to us to appreciate its full significance. We do not know of any pressure brought to bear upon the declarant(s) to make this declaration, and we believe it is made by his/her (their) own wish and solely on behalf of the better interests of their child(ren) about to be born.

_____   _____
Witness   Witness

NEW SECTION. Sec. 12. Short title. This Act may be cited as the Severely Defective Children's Euthanasia Act of 19_____.

NEW SECTION. Sec. 13. Severability. If any provision of this Act, or its application to any person or circumstance is held invalid, the remainder of the Act, or the application of the provision to other persons or circumstances is not affected.

NEW SECTION. Sec. 14. Captions and section headings. Captions and section headings used in this Act shall not constitute any part of law.

Notes

1. The following is a set of provisions for legislation that might be enacted. What is needed is a comprehensive statute that fully remedies the law's defective premise while simultaneously creating procedures that ensure the achievement of the desired ends and that ensure against abuse and otherwise provide protection.

2. I thank Mr. Gary Reid, Assistant Code Reviser, Statute Law Committee, State of Washington, for revising my proposed statute and putting it into the style commonly used by the National Conference of Commissioners on Uniform State Law. Mr. Reid is not to be held responsible for any of the substantive defects in the proposed statute, although there are fewer because of his excellent work.

Thomas Harvey

Annotated Bibliography

BOOKS

Cummin, William. *The Proofs of Infanticide Considered: Including Dr. Hunter's Tract on Child Murder, With Illustrative Notes; and a Summary of the Present State of Medico-Legal Knowledge on the Subject.* London: Wilson and Son, 1836.

This book consists of three distinct parts. The first part is Dr. Hunter's tract on child murder entitled, "On the Uncertainty of the Signs of Murder, in the Case of Bastard Children." In his paper Dr. Hunter expresses two main themes concerning infanticide. The first theme is a very sympathetic and compassionate plea for merciful treatment of those who commit this crime. Dr. Hunter blames society for causing mothers to be outcasts and, thereby, bringing about the depression that causes the act of infanticide to occur. The second theme Dr. Hunter expresses is the medical pitfalls of legally proving child murder in these cases. The second and third parts of the book consist of Dr. Cummin's reply to Dr. Hunter's paper. In the second part, "Notes and Illustrations," Dr. Cummin goes through Dr. Hunter's paper, points out where he believes Dr. Hunter's paper was inconsistent or incomplete, and questions many of Dr. Hunter's conclusions. In the third part of the book, "Summary of Medico-Legal Facts Connected with Infanticide," Dr. Cummin expresses what he feels is a complete treatise on the medical and legal aspects of infanticide. He tries to show that legally the medical proof that infanticide has occurred is not as dubious a proof as Dr. Hunter has asserted.

Jonsen, Albert R., and Garland, Michael J., eds. *Ethics of Newborn Intensive Care*. Health Policy Program, School of Medicine, University of California and Berkeley. San Francisco: Institute of Governmental Studies, University of California, 1976.

A comprehensive investigation of the complex dilemmas that must be confronted and resolved in newborn intensive care. This work confronts these dilemmas in a straightforward manner from as many divergent disciplines as is possible. The book initially considers the current state of neonatal intensive care from a medical viewpoint, presents three case histories of neonatal intensive care, presents a historical perspective of neonatal medicine and the quality of life, and investigates the mental development of the survivors of neonatal intensive care. The ethical issues involved in neonatal intensive care are then discussed from various viewpoints. Divergent views on the ethics of infant euthanasia are immediately followed by the presentation of a moral policy to help those persons involved make life and death decisions in the intensive care nursery.

PERIODICALS

Arboleda-Florez, Julio. "Infanticide. Some Medicolegal Considerations." *Canadian Psychiatric Association Journal* 20, no. 1 (February 1975): 55-60.

In this paper the author initially defines neonaticide (the murder of a child by its mother within the first twenty-four hours postpartum) and infanticide (the murder of a child by its mother within the first year of life). He then reviews various legal practices concerning infanticide in the past. He points out that the traditional legal definitions regard neonaticide and infanticide as identical crimes. The author further reviews the medical data available with respect to the etiology of this homicidal act by a mother. He concludes his paper by stating that most infanticides are committed for altruistic reasons, while most neonaticides are committed because the child is not wanted. The author charges that the law, in differentiating between murder and infanticide while not differentiating between neonaticide and infanticide, is being discriminatory and that this legal distinction should, therefore, be abolished.

Bender, Lauretta. "Psychiatric Mechanism in Child Murders." *Journal of Nervous and Mental Disease* 80 (1934): 32-47.

The author uses a case study approach to investigate and summarize what she believes to be the causes for, and the reactions to, acts of infanticide. The study is limited to acts of murder where the children are not infants and where the mothers are married. The author concludes that child murder by parents is a suicidal act as a result of identification processes.

Brozovsky, Morris, and Falit, Harvey. "Neonaticide: Clinical and Psychodynamic Consideration." *American Academy of Child Psychiatry Journal* 10 (October 1971): 673-683.

A psychological study, using two test cases and histories previously recorded, to show the severe mental anxiety of mothers who have committed neonaticide. The study excludes "those infrequent cases in which a psychopathic mother plans, in full consciousness, to murder her unwanted infant." The authors identify the following characteristics of the act of neonaticide: most of the women are unmarried and facing societal rejection; these women predominately use the form of denial to release their tension; so intense is the denial of pregnancy that in a vast number of cases these women can inhibit the physical manifestations of pregnancy. The authors conclude that, "It is our hypothesis that neonaticide stems from the ego disorganization which occurs when denial, so tenaciously clung to during the pregnancy and delivery, is made no longer tenable by the actual birth of the child."

Button, Jesse H., and Reivich, Ronald S. "Obsessions of Infanticide." *Archives of General Psychiatry* 27 (August 1971): 235-240.

A psychological study of infanticidal obsession reviewing forty-two cases. The infanticidal obsession was a clinically prominent feature of the patient's psychopathologic condition. Among the conclusions of the authors is the following significant statement: "Diagnostically, a reasonably strong case could be made for classifying all of the men in the schizophrenic category." The authors also indicated that for women the hormonal secretions (prior to menstruation, menopause, birth, and after birth) cause depression that, in the eyes of these doctors, is the major cause of infanticide.

Culliton, Barbara J. "Intensive Care for Newborns: Are There Times to Pull the Plug?" *Science* 188 (April 1975): 133-134.

A summary of the ethical dilemmas discussed and the moral policies adopted at a conference in California, where the problems considered were the ethical issues in newborn intensive care. The article concludes by listing the statements of this moral policy.

Duff, Raymond S., and Campbell, A. G. M. "Moral and Ethical Dilemmas in the Special-Care Nursery." *New England Journal of Medicine* 289, no. 17 (October 25, 1973): 890-894.

An article that investigates the very difficult decisions that concern the life, death, and quality of life of severely deformed and handicapped infants. These decisions are investigated from the various points of reference of the infant, the infant's family, the professional staff, and society. The moral and ethical issues are investigated and confronted without regard for what is legal or illegal. The position of the authors is, "If working out these dilemmas in ways such as those we suggest is in violation of the law, we believe the law should be changed."

Fletcher, John. "Abortion, Euthanasia, and Care of Defective Newborns." *New England Journal of Medicine* 292, no. 2 (January 9, 1975): 75-77.

The author clearly presents two polarized ethical positions concerning the compatibility of the abortion of defective fetuses and the euthanasia of defective infants. The first position disapprovingly equates genetically indicated abortion with infanticide, while the second position approvingly equates the selective euthanasia of defective infants with abortion. The author then strives to establish his ethical position, which accepts the abortion of a seriously defective fetus but rejects euthanasia for defective newborns.

———. "Attitudes Toward Defective Newborns." *Hastings Center Studies* 2, no. 1 (January 1974): 21-32.

This paper investigates the shape and meaning of developing attitudes toward the congenitally abnormal newborn infant. There is a historical introduction that conveys the attitudes and actions of past peoples towards defective newborns. The author then writes of the present attitudes of parents and health professionals. He speaks of the initially negative attitudes of the parents, and possibly the health professionals, towards the defective newborn being gradually overcome and built into a more complex attitude of acceptance. The author outlines this process of change and many of the contributing factors that influence both the degree of initial rejection of the infant and the flexibility or inflexibility of this rejection. The author concludes his paper by advancing the thesis that new developments in genetics (amniocentesis techniques) will cause our attitudes towards genetically defective infants to become harsher and more inflexible.

Jonsen, A. R.; Phibbs, R. H.; Tooley, W. H.; and Garland, M. J. "Critical Issues in Newborn Intensive Care: A Conference Report and Policy Proposal." *Pediatrics* 55, no. 6 (June 1975): 756-768.

> A paper that describes a conference, the purpose of which was to consider the ethical problems raised by neonatal intensive care. The conference brought together twenty persons from the various disciplines of medicine, nursing, law, sociology, psychology, ethics, economics, social work, anthropology, and the news media. The paper is divided into two parts and two appendixes. Part one of the paper summarizes the materials presented to the participants: five illustrative cases, papers presented upon the major considerations, and four clinical questions. All the discussion and argument is, of course, not presented but a consensus of the participant's opinions is given in Appendix B—the responses to the four clinical questions. Part two of the paper presents a moral policy that hopefully reflects the consensus of opinion of the twenty participants and defines the terms moral value, responsibility, duty, and interest. Appendix A is a list of the conference participants.

Harder, Thoger. "The Psychopathology of Infanticide." *ACTA Psychiatrica Scandinavica* 43 (1967): 196-245.

> A precise and thorough psychological study of acts, or attempted acts, of infanticide. The author reviews past studies, presents a complete psychiatric case history of nineteen persons charged with killing, or the attempted killing, of their children, and then examines each case in the light of previous studies. In particular, the author presents a discussion of the diagnosis of endogenous contra psychogenic depression and a strong criticism of the concept that infanticide can be altruistic in nature.

Heymann, Philip B., and Holtz, Sara. "The Severely Defective Newborn: The Dilemma and the Decision Process." *Public Policy* 23, no. 4 (Fall 1975): 381-417.

> A clear and comprehensive explanation of the manner in which

the judicial system functions to define social norms of conduct. The authors first explain, in broad social terms, the limitations of the judicial system, with respect to mandating social behavior. They then narrow the scope of the paper to define reasonable treatment for patients in general, and for infants with severe spina bifida, in particular. The authors confront, within a legal framework, many of the most crucial medical and ethical dilemmas initiated by the severely defective newborn. Considered within the legal context are the dilemmas presented by passive and active euthanasia for defective newborns and a possible redefining of personhood.

Kellum, Barbara A. "Infanticide in England in the Later Middle Ages." *History of Childhood Quarterly* 1, no. 3 (Winter 1974): 367-388.

The author traces the history of infanticide in England in the late Middle Ages by investigating sex ratios and the concern of the church with child murder. She concludes that infanticide was common, that it was motivated by poverty and illegitimacy, and was an accepted means of population control.

Kelsey, Beverly. "An Interview with Dr. Raymond S. Duff: Which Infants Should Live? Who Should Decide?" *Hastings Center Report* (April 1975): 5-8.

Dr. Duff's responses to a series of very difficult and provoking questions related to the birth of a severely deformed infant. In responding to these questions, Dr. Duff gives a description of the decision-making process that families experience in attempting to resolve the dilemmas initiated by the birth of a severely deformed infant. The ethical distinction between allowing the infant to die and actively killing the infant is commented upon by Dr. Duff and Sister Margaret Farley.

Langer, William L. "Checks on Population Growth: 1750-1850." *Scientific American* (1972): 91-100.

The author states that the population of Europe nearly doubled in this period, and maintains that without the checks of celibacy and infanticide the population would have grown considerably more. Initially investigated are the laws and attitudes that made celibacy an important check on population. The author then confronts the reader with evidence that indicates that infanticide was a widespread and much accepted form of population control despite strict legal penalties and church condemnation.

————. "Further Notes on the History of Infanticide." *History of Childhood Quarterly* 2, no. 1 (Summer 1974): 129-134.

The author investigates the history of the practice of infanticide in the ancient Roman and Greek cultures, in Europe during the Middle Ages, and in China, Japan, and India. Supportive data is scanty and inductive logic is used in places where more quantitative data is unobtainable, but the conclusion is that the practice of infanticide as a population control was quite common due to socio-economic conditions.

————. "Infanticide: A Historical Survey." *History of Childhood Quarterly* 1, no. 3 (Winter 1974): 363-365.

The author maintains that throughout history infanticide has been an accepted method of population and quality of population control. He states clearly the reason he feels an understanding of the history of infanticide is significant: ". . . in these days of world population crisis there can hardly be a more important historical question than that of the chronically superfluous population growth and the methods by which humanity has dealt with it." The author begins his survey of the history of infanticide by mentioning the frequency of its use for population and quality of population control in ancient China, Hellenistic Greece, and the Roman Empire. The author quickly narrows the scope of the paper to deal more specifically with the European history of infanticide, with special emphasis directed towards France and England. He devotes much of his paper to France and England in specifying the frequency of infanticide, the manner in which this child murder was achieved, and the massive efforts in these countries to curb its practice.

Lorber, J. "Results of Treatment of Myelomeningocele: An Analysis of 524 Unselected Cases, with Special Reference to Possible Selection for Treatment." *Developmental Medicine and Child Neurology* 13 (1971): 279-303.

This paper is a statistical survey of 524 unselected cases of mye-lomeningocele. The author himself summarizes his work best in the following quotations that respectively state the problem that the paper investigates, the purposes of the paper, the limita-tions placed upon the paper, and the conclusions that the author draws from his paper: 1. "It is felt by some that all affected infants should be operated upon even if it is certain that many survivors will suffer from multiple handicaps. This policy is a source of anxiety to others who consider it wrong to treat those infants whose predictable quality of life would be poor." 2. "It would be of considerable value if one could foretell from sim-ple physical signs present on the first day of life the likely future of a baby if he were untreated, and compare this with his chances if he were given the total care as is known today. This paper at-tempts to give such data which may serve as a guide to those called upon to advise and deal with infants born with myelomen-ingocele." 3. "This paper does not deal with the effect such a child (spina bifida) had on family life and finances, nor does it deal with the effect on the hospital services, schools, and the community. It is not concerned with the tremendous cost in-volved. All these are important and will be dealt with elsewhere, but their consideration should not cloud the main issue: the in-terest of the patient." 4. "It is possible to forecast from a purely clinical assessment with accuracy the minimal degree of future han-dicap in an individual even if it is impossible to forecast the maximum degree of disability which he may suffer, if he sur-vives. Even with careful selection there will be some children who will be severely handicapped."

McCormick, Richard A. "To Save or Let Die: The Dilemma of Modern Medicine." *Journal of the American Medical Association* 229, no. 2 (July 8, 1974): 172-176.

The author addresses himself to one of the most troublesome ethical dilemmas of modern medicine, the severely defective newborn. He points out that the sophistication of modern medicine has forced an awesome responsibility upon us, the making of quality-of-life judgments. The author maintains that with increased knowledge comes increased responsibility, and we must not evade it. Like it or not, we must establish broad guidelines that will help parents and doctors make these difficult quality-of-life decisions. Ethically, he argues against life being the ultimate good to be cherished and maintained absolutely. The author maintains that life in and of itself is not an absolute good but is only a limited good, in that it is a necessary condition for the achievement of the higher values—meaningful relation potential.

McDermaid, G., and Winkler, E. G. "Psychopathology of Infanticide." *Journal of Clinical and Experimental Psychopathology* 16, no. 1 (March 1955): 22-41.

A psychological paper that investigates common motivations in cases of infanticide, hoping to be able to recognize the potentialities toward infanticide and, thereby, recommend proper treatment to alleviate the conditions that motivate an act of child murder. The authors pursued a case history approach of twelve cases and generalized the results. The majority of these patients expressed depression with suicidal tendencies. The authors concluded that, "The depressive state weakens the ego functions, suicidal tendencies become manifest, and the child that is considered as part of the person's own body is the victim of self-destruction."

Melges, Frederick T. "Postpartum Psychiatric Syndromes." *Psychosomatic Medicine* 30, no. 1 (1968): 95-108.

An excellent psychological paper which tries to determine why there is a four- to fivefold increase in the risk of mental illness for women during the first three months after the birth of an infant. One hundred patients in the sample were chosen according to two criteria: the onset of psychiatric illness occurred during the time period spanning one month prepartum to three months postpartum, and the psychiatrist in charge of the patients deemed childbearing to be a significant factor in the onset of mental illness. After extensive testing the author drew the following conclusions: 1. Lack of difference between these patients and control subjects in performance using EEG, serial-7 and digit-span tests militated against the existence of a toxic delirious state. 2. Hormonal changes may make some women more vulnerable, but since three patients became bewildered shortly after adoption of an infant, it appears that the psychological conflict over mothering can precipitate a confusional syndrome in the absence of postpartum physiological changes. 3. The author postulated that the high incidence of confusion most likely stems from identity diffusion, centering around a conflict in assuming the mothering role. 4. In the majority of patients, this conflict appeared to result from the patient's repudiation of their own mothers as adequate models.

Myers, Steven A. "Maternal Filicide." *American Journal Disabled Child* 120 (December 1970): 534-536.

A survey of thirty-five instances in which a mother was responsible for the death of her preadolescent child. In the vast majority of cases, the mothers were judged to be psychotic at the time of their child's death. The author maintains that most of these women were suffering from psychotic depression and a number were schizophrenic. He concludes that recognition of the symptoms of these illnesses is the initial step in the prevention of maternal filicide.

Robertson, John A. "Involuntary Euthanasia of Defective Newborns: A Legal Analysis." *Stanford Law Review* 27 (January 1975): 213-269.

This significant paper deals primarily with the legal aspects of involuntary passive euthanasia of defective infants. It is not possible to summarize the purpose and content of this paper more concisely than does the author himself: "This article analyzes the criminal liability of the parties involved in the decision to withhold treatment from defective infants and attempts a reasoned evaluation of current legal policy. It takes the position that under existing law parents, physicians and hospital staff commit several crimes in withholding care, and that on the whole, with few exceptions, criminal liability may be both desirable and morally compelled. It argues further that a principled case for nonliability can be made only if we are prepared to establish a legislative definition of a narrow class of persons from whom care justifiably can be withheld, and if procedural safeguards to limit the possibility of arbitrary decisions are instituted. Depending on one's view of the issue, present criminal sanctions should be enforced more fully, or legislation permitting nontreatment should be enacted."

————., and Fost, Norman. "Passive Euthanasia of Defective Newborn Infants: Legal Considerations." *Journal of Pediatrics* 88, no. 5 (May 1976): 883-889.

A paper that outlines the legal responsibilities of parents, physicians, nurses, and hospital administrators that elect to allow, or are simply aware of, the passive euthanasia of defective newborn infants. The authors argue that withholding treatment for defective newborn infants has become widespread and, although much ethical debate concerning this practice has occurred, discussion of this practice within a social context and the appropriateness of current law has been minimal. The authors define and clarify homicide by omission, first and second degree murder, involuntary manslaughter, child abuse statutes, and what it means to be an accessory. The authors then explain how parents, physicians, nurses, and hospital administrators may be legally liable for a number of these offenses for their involvement in the passive euthanasia of a defective infant. The authors further state that although there has not been any criminal prosecution, as yet, for the nontreatment of a defective newborn, that this prosecution is sure to occur, if only to clarify the law. The authors encourage all those involved to follow due process to formulate a legal policy. "By claiming the right to act in ignorance or defiance of existing legal principles and statutes the physician, parent, nurse, or hospital administration claims a right he would not ascribe to others."

Rodenburg, Martin. "Child Murder by Depressed Parents." *Canadian Psychiatric Association Journal* 16, no. 1 (February 1971): 41-48.

The author reviews past surveys and presents statistical research related to the murder of children by depressed parents. The stated purpose of the paper is to identify symptoms that lead to child murder so that the early recognition of these symptoms might lead to the prevention of this crime. The author concludes that when a depressive illness is superimposed upon a constellation of parental factors, which can be recognized, a child is most vulnerable to this type of crime.

Shaw, Anthony. "Dilemmas of 'Informed Consent' in Children." *New England Journal of Medicine* 289, no. 17 (October 25, 1973): 885-890.

Traditionally, patients have at least one legal right—that of informed consent. This paper addresses itself to the inherent legal and ethical dilemmas presented when that patient is a minor. The author discusses problem areas of informed consent involving infants and minors, including religious freedom. The author reaches the following conclusion: "Once the physician has discharged his obligation fully to inform an adult mentally competent patient, that patient may then accept or reject the proposed treatment, or, indeed, may refuse any and all treatment as he sees fit. But if the patient is a minor, a parental decision rejecting recommended treatment is subject to review when physicians or society disagree with that decision."

Smith, G., and Smith, E. "Selection for Treatment in Spina Bifida Cystica." *British Medical Journal* 27 (October 1973): 189-197.

The authors outline the program of selective treatment of spina bifida cystica employed at the Royal Children's Hospital, Melbourne, Victoria, Australia. In the context of this paper the mortality rate of these infants, the quality of life of the survivors, and the implications of both of these factors, with respect to the future selection process, are discussed. No early surgery was given 27 percent of these infants and their mortality rate was understandably high. Basically, the program presented recommends immediate repair of the sac in most low lesions, defers treatment in high lesions, and employs reevaluation of all the survivors of this later group at one month and later for possible active treatment.

Trexler, Richard C. "Infanticide in Florence: New Sources and First Results." *History of Childhood Quarterly* 1, no. 1 (1973): 98-116.

A historical paper that presents two pieces of quantifiable evidence that strongly suggests that infanticide was a fact of life in Florence during the fifteenth and sixteenth centuries.

Working Party of the New Castle Regional Hospital Board. "Ethics of Selective Treatment of Spina Bifida." *The Lancet* 1 (January, 11, 1975): 85-88.

The Working Party of the New Castle Regional Hospital Board addressed itself to the ethical dilemma initiated by the birth of an infant with spina bifida. The Working Party felt that ethical problems in medicine arise when normal guiding principles appear to be in conflict. In this particular case, the conflict is between the principle that human life is sacred and the principle that any decision requires an estimate of the balance of suffering and happiness for those concerned in the decision. The discussion of this conflict, in the particular case of an infant with spina bifida, drew the following conclusions: the physician has no ethical obligation to treat cases in which the likely benefits are very dubious; although nontreatment (passive euthanasia) is an alternative, active euthanasia is not; and the long term aims of medical research in this field must be to recognize the causes of these abnormalities and to remove them.

Contributors

PETER BLACK

Dr. Black, now in neurosurgical training at the Massachusetts General Hospital, is also finishing a philosophy dissertation at Georgetown University on the differences between killing and letting die.

RICHARD BRANDT

R. B. Brandt was educated at Denison, Cambridge, and Yale universities, taught at Swarthmore College, and is now professor at the University of Michigan. He has authored *Ethical Theory, Hopi Ethics,* and (forthcoming) *A Theory of the Good and the Right,* and articles in the journals, especially on utilitarianism.

JOHN DONNELLY

John Donnelly took his Ph.D. in philosophy at Brown University and is currently associate professor of philosophy and chairman of the department at the University of San Diego. He is the editor of *Logical Analysis and Contemporary Theism, Conscience,* and *Language, Meta-*

physics, and Death.

RAYMOND S. DUFF

Dr. Duff is professor of pediatrics at Yale University. For most of his professional life, his time has been divided between caring for children (including the counselling of parents) and research and teaching in behavioral aspects of health.

JOSEPH FLETCHER

Robert Treat Paine Professor of Social Ethics, Emeritus, Episcopal Theological School, Dr. Fletcher is visiting professor of biomedical ethics, School of Medicine, University of Virginia, and Senior Fellow in Biomedical Ethics, University of Texas Graduate School of Biomedical Sciences.

THOMAS HARVEY

Thomas Harvey studies philosophy and is a teacher of mathematics at Fredonia High School, Fredonia, New York.

IMMANUEL JAKOBOVITS

Dr. Jakobovits is Chief Rabbi of the United Hebrew Congregations of the British Commonwealth of Nations and President of the Institute of Judaism and Medicine, Jerusalem. He is the author of *Jewish Medical Ethics* (1959, 1974) and *Jewish Law Faces Modern Problems* (1965).

EIKE-HENNER W. KLUGE

Eike-Henner W. Kluge is associate professor of philosophy, University of Victoria. Other publications in related areas of ethics include *The Practice of Death* (1975) and "The Right to Life of Potential Persons" (*Dalhousie Law Journal*, 1977). He is currently working on a book on euthanasia.

MARVIN KOHL

Dr. Kohl is professor of philosophy at the State University of New York at Fredonia. He is the author of *The Morality of Killing* (1974) and editor of *Beneficent Euthanasia* (1975).

JOSEPH MARGOLIS

Joseph Margolis is professor of philosophy, Temple University. His most recent book is *Persons and Mind* (1977). His *Art and Philosophy* is forthcoming.

KAREN METZLER

Ms. Metzler was born with spina bifida and other problems. She has nearly grown up in the hospital, having undergone an estimated fifty-eight operations, including an amputation of her right leg. She is a twenty-six-year-old psychology major, who graduated magna cum laude from Baldwin Wallace College, and who presently works as a health care consultant and lecturer.

ARVAL A. MORRIS

Professor of law at the University of Washington in Seattle, where Dr. Morris has been actively involved with problems posed for the law by recent advances in biomedical technology. He is the author of *The Constitution and American Education* (1974) and articles in various journals.

STEPHEN NATHANSON

Stephen Nathanson teaches philosophy at Northeastern University and has written on Locke, scepticism, rationality, and John Barth.

ANTHONY SHAW

Anthony Shaw, M.D. is professor of surgery and pediatrics at the University of Virginia School of Medicine in Charlottesville. Author of "Doctor, Do We Have a Choice?" in the *New York Times Magazine*, Dr. Shaw has written widely for lay and professional periodicals on medical decision making and the severely impaired newborn.

BRANDT F. STEELE

Professor of psychiatry at University of Colorado Medical Center and psychiatrist at the National Center for Prevention and Treatment of Child Abuse and Neglect, Denver. He is a training analyst at Denver Psychoanalytic Institute and the author of many articles on child abuse and violence.

LEONARD WEBER

Leonard J. Weber is an associate professor of Religious Studies at Mercy College of Detroit. He received his Ph.D. from McMaster University. He is the author of *Who Shall Live? The Dilemma of Severely Handicapped Children and Its Meaning for Other Moral Questions* (1976).

GLANVILLE WILLIAMS

Rouse Ball Professor of English Law in the University Cambridge and Honorary Bencher of the Middle Temple, London. Professor Williams is President of the Abortion Law Reform Association, London, and author of numerous works including *The Sanctity of Life and the Criminal Law* (1957).

LAILA WILLIAMSON

Ms. Williamson, an anthropologist, is curatorial assistant in the department of anthropology of the American Museum of Natural History.